For Churchill Livingstone:

Commissioning Editor: Susan Young
Development Editor: Catherine Jackson
Project Manager: Joannah Duncan
Designer: Judith Wright
Illustration Manager: Bruce Hogarth

Teaching For Health
Third Edition

Revised by
Alice M. Kiger

BA, MA, MSc, PhD, RN, DipN, RCNT, RNT
Director, Centre for Advanced Studies in Nursing,
University of Aberdeen, Aberdeen, UK

First Edition by Lyn Coutts and Leslie Hardy
Second Edition Revised by Alice M. Kiger

Foreword by
Leslie Hardy

BN, MCSNEd, PhD
Formerly Nurse

Lyn Coutts Mitchell

BScSocSci, MMedSci, RGN, RGM, RSCN
Formerly Chief Executive, National Board
for Nursing, Midwifery and Health Visiting,
Scotland

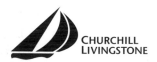
CHURCHILL
LIVINGSTONE

EDINBURGH LONDON NEW YORK OXFORD PHILADELPHIA ST LOUIS SYDNEY TORONTO 2004

CHURCHILL LIVINGSTONE
An imprint of Elsevier Limited

© Pearson Professional Limited 1985
© Churchill Livingstone 1995
© 2004, Elsevier Limited. All rights reserved.

First edition 1985
Second edition 1995
Third edition 2004
   Reprinted 2007

ISBN 978 0 443 07298 7

British Library Cataloguing in Publication Data
A catalogue record for this book is available from the British Library.

Library of Congress Cataloging in Publication Data
A catalog record for this book is available from the Library of Congress.

Note
Knowledge and best practice in this field are constantly changing. As new research and experience broaden our knowledge, changes in practice, treatment and drug therapy may become necessary or appropriate. readers are advised to check the most current information provided (i) on procedures featured or (ii) by the manufacturer of each product to be administered, to verify the recommended dose or formula, the method and duration of administration, and contraindications. It is the responsibility of the practitioner, relying on their own experience and knowledge of the patient, to make diagnoses, to determine dosages and the best treatment for each individual patient, and to take all appropriate safety precautions. To the fullest extent of the law, neither the publisher nor the authors assumes any liability for any injury and/or damage.

The Publisher

Printed in China

Contents

Section One: THEORETICAL UNDERPINNINGS

1 Health and its promotion   3

The meaning of health; Planning for health; Measuring health: mortality statistics, morbidity statistics, population statistics; Current ill health in Britain: mortality, morbidity; Some international comparisons; Positive views of health; Health education and health promotion; Ethical issues in health promotion; References.

2 Health education concepts and practice   29

Health education approaches and models: the information-giving (medical) model, the educational model, the propaganda (media) model, the enabling (community development) model, the political action model, reflection on the models; health education services in the United Kingdom: national organizations; An international look at health education/promotion: Canada, Australia, South Africa; Nurses as health teachers; Teaching for health; References.

3 Learning about health   63

Ideas about learning and teaching: defining teaching, defining learning, the teaching–learning process; Theoretical considerations relevant to learning: learning theories, domains of learning, levels of learning, motivation for learning, the relationship of memory to learning, learning styles, the adult as learner, readiness to learn, fostering learning; References.

4 Therapeutic and persuasive communication   83

Therapeutic communication; The communication process: elements of communication, the dynamic of communication; Techniques of therapeutic communication: questioning, listening and the use of silence, interview types and techniques; Persuasive communication: the link between beliefs, attitudes and behaviour, theories relevant to the formation of attitudes; Factors affecting communication and persuasion: the setting, the nurse, the patient or client, the message; References.

5 Teaching techniques and aids   109

Teaching for understanding and recall; Teaching for skills learning; Encouraging affective learning; Teaching methods: the lecture method, group work, demonstration, role play; Choosing teaching techniques and aids: choice of technique, choice of aid; References.

Section Two: THE PROCESS OF HEALTH TEACHING

Section Three: ISSUES IN HEALTH TEACHING

Preface

There have been many changes in the health care systems, and in the education of health professionals in the United Kingdom and elsewhere, since the first edition of *Teaching for Health* was published in 1985, and change has continued apace since the second edition of 1995. The increased emphasis on health rather than illness, and the transfer of a growing proportion of care from the acute to the community setting, mean that this book's subject matter remains highly relevant.

The aims of this third edition are unchanged from the two previous editions. Information has been brought up to date, and the content has been modified to reflect the current context of health. In addition to focusing on health teaching as it applies within the UK, an effort has been made to reflect aspects of international health concerns.

The organisation of the book's content is unchanged from the second edition. The book is divided into three sections. The first contains a range of theoretical underpinnings to the practice of health teaching. The second covers the four phases of the health teaching process. The third section revisits the underpinnings of the process and offers a chapter that addresses research relevant to health teaching and another that reflects on a number of ethical and theoretical issues of particular concern to nurses, midwives and other professionals who act as health teachers.

Student activities are included within each chapter (see 'To the student' and 'To the teacher' on the following pages) to enhance the practical use of the book, and 'Questions for review and reflection' are offered at the end of the book.

It is hoped that this third edition of Teaching for Health will continue to suit the needs of students of nursing, midwifery and other health care professions in both pre-registration programmes and post-registration or postgraduate programmes. It is further hoped that teachers of health professionals will find the book equally helpful in their support of students who are learning to 'teach for health'.

Alice M. Kiger, 2004

Foreword

The continuing need for health teaching and, therefore, this third edition of *Teaching for Health*, is evidence that nurses believe not only that they play a crucial role in helping people to learn about health, but also that they need to persist in working at reducing stubborn inequities in health. What is novel today is a growing hunger in the public to know more, to participate more fully in health decisions and to practise healthy behaviour. Nurses are the most accessible of all health professionals who can fulfil the teaching role and those who make health policy are recognising this fact more and more.

This latest edition of *Teaching for Health* arrives almost 20 years after the first edition (1985). The period has been replete with health promotion/teaching and health marketing by governments, health professionals and other agencies. Those now entering the nursing profession have lived from birth through an intensive, sustained and organised period of health teaching and will be more than able to reflect on what has had an impact on their personal health decision-making. Nurse educators can draw on this richness of experience to make student learning more meaningful.

The complexity of health teaching has grown, with information flowing from many fields. For example, we know that personality is well developed by the age of three years and is resistant to change, although some behaviours can be modified with a great deal of effort. Does this mean that health behaviours are also set by this early age? What would such information mean for health teaching?

A recent book by Barbara Strauch (2003), *The Primal Teen: What the New Discoveries About the Teenage Brain Tell Us About Our Kids* (New York: Doubleday), reports on research which found that the prefrontal cortex, the area of the brain responsible for reasoning, risk assessment and impulse control, develops last in adolescents, sometimes as late as into their twenties. These findings have major implications for parents, teachers and health professionals working with teenagers. Alice Kiger emphasizes the need for a rational plan based on 'the best available evidence' (p.8) and carries this significant advice through the book. The roles of evidence-based practice, evaluation and research from nursing and other appropriate fields can only enhance health teaching.

One of the major changes in society since the early 1980s has been the widespread acceptance of the Internet. Access to health information is easy, and support groups for various health concerns are available or can be set up quickly. However, users must be educated to sort the good advice from the bad, to use trustworthy sites and avoid those selling bogus products or advice. When an Internet site claimed that aspartame, an artificial sweetener, was responsible for all sorts of health problems, the article was widely read and reproduced in print without any checking of its validity, in spite of the fact that an official from the Food and Drug Administration in the United States quickly composed a response which refuted most of the 'facts' in the piece. Another concern is that the commercialization of health is growing because of the Internet. The whole world is now an accessible market and vendors of easy cures have been quick to realize the potential and have perfected their marketing skills. How do consumers choose when they are innundated with conflicting health messages from multiple sources? Health teachers are needed for interpretation and guidance.

Health teachers today face many new factors influencing health behaviour. In North

America, school board trustees have signed contracts with international soft drink companies to install pop machines in schools. This raises funds for school activities as well as profit for the companies, but at a cost – increased intake of junk calories which contribute to childhood obesity. For the trustees, fund-raising took precedence over health. Furthermore, children are particularly susceptible to advertising and peer pressure and will frequently choose popular foods over healthy alternatives. Health teaching is more complex than ever before.

Western politicians tend to make short-term promises tied to election times. This means short-term planning and a focus on issues which can be quickly resolved and get positive attention; a direct contrast to the long-term planning needed for health promotion and teaching and the evaluation of any teaching. Alice Kiger makes it clear that health teaching cannot be sidelined but is an integral part of health care in all its facets. Nurses and midwives must be ready with evidence to argue their case to the advantage of the public. This textbook offers valuable information on teaching concepts, approaches and issues, as well as considering the wider remit of health teachers to study, assess and influence government health policy.

Leslie K. Hardy
Lyn Coutts Mitchell
2004

Acknowledgements

The author wishes to thank colleagues in the Centre for Advanced Studies in Nursing at the University of Aberdeen (Helen Robertson, Vanora Hundley and Sally Lawton) for their patience during the revision of this book, and especially for their hard work and support during what turned out to be an exceedingly busy period for us all. Additional thanks to Sally for assistance with early literature searching.

Sincere thanks to the staff at Elsevier for their excellent assistance during the preparation of the book, particularly to Catherine Jackson, who has been especially patient and supportive during the latter stages of writing.

Particular thanks to the stoma care nurses, Christine Finlay, Marion Tierney Strachen and Alison Paterson, and to Eloise Pearson, clinical nurse manager for ambulatory care, theatres and general surgery, all in NHS Grampian. They provided expert advice for the updating of sections of Chapter 8.

Special thanks to Tony for his ever-faithful encouragement, helpful ideas and tolerant listening, and for his willingness to do more than his share of the housework.

Finally, a particular note of thanks to Lyn Mitchell (née Coutts) and Leslie Hardy, authors of the first edition. I hope they will feel that this third edition is maintaining the tradition they established with the first.

Alice M. Kiger, 2004

To the teacher

This book can be used as a central course text, or it can be part of a recommended reading list for a course on health or health education/promotion.

The 'Activities' provided in each chapter can be used selectively according to the aims of the course and the students' needs. If the book is being used as a central course text, the teacher can select the activities that are most suited to the level and experience of the students. Activities can be carried out either in or outside the class. Students may, of course, choose to do the activities on their own.

The 'Questions for review and reflection' at the end of the book might be used as the basis for classroom discussions or seminars, or students can be assigned selected questions to do on their own. No answer key is provided, as many of these questions do not have 'correct' answers, and for those that do, the answers can be found within the content of the book. It is suggested that teachers provide students with the opportunity to discuss their responses, if questions have been assigned for out-of-class work.

To the student

This book is arranged so that you can read it as a textbook or interact with it as a basis for active learning. An interactive approach is preferred by the author.

Throughout the book you will find 'Activities' to support the material in each chapter. These activities are intended to stimulate deeper levels of learning, something more than merely committing the material to memory. You can carry them out as part of class activities, if directed to do so by your tutor or lecturer, or you can carry them out on your own, with a classmate, or with a group of classmates. You do not have to do them all. Some can be quite time-consuming. If you are using the book on your own, you may find you do not have enough time, so you should select from the activities according to your own needs. Even if you do not have time to carry out the activities as described, you may find it helpful to read them and to reflect on the ideas they contain.

At the end of the book you will find a set of 'Questions for review and reflection'. As with the activities, you may choose from these to suit your needs. No 'answer key' has been provided, as many of the questions or problems do not have single correct answers. They are meant to stretch your ability to reason, solve problems and think creatively. For those that do have specific correct answers, these can be found within the book's contents, and searching for them should be a useful exercise that will help reinforce your learning.

1 THEORETICAL UNDERPINNINGS

SECTION CONTENTS

Health and its promotion

THE MEANING OF HEALTH

Before considering how to 'teach for health', it is important to consider the meaning of health. Notice how the concept has been phrased here. 'The meaning of health' might be understood in two different ways: it could be seen to imply a definition, but it could also be taken to refer to the subjective perception of 'health' by an individual person. The latter sense indicates one of the truths about health: it is not an objective fact, it is a subjectively understood concept. Thus it may justifiably be said that what health is, is a matter of opinion.

In the Judeo-Christian tradition, health meant wholeness; it contained the idea of blessedness or salvation (Mercer 2000). Greek and Roman ideas on health centred on the concept of well-being. Health and happiness were closely related (Kirsten 2001). In Islamic thinking, health is seen as a state of dynamic equilibrium in which the body functions normally (Khayat 1997) and is a matter of balance relating to both body and soul (Abu Reidah 2003).

Many modern definitions reflect a synthesis of such ideas. It is often said that health has three dimensions which are in delicate balance: the physical, mental and social dimensions. In recent years a fourth dimension, that of spiritual health, has been added. Upset in any one of these areas can affect the others. For instance, it is common to suffer a feeling of depression along with a physical illness, and it is common for a person suffering depression to experience physical symptoms. So there exists the idea that health is a state of balance between various aspects of life. When these aspects are in balance, we experience a quality of life we call health.

Katherine Mansfield (Savary et al 1970) has described what that quality of life meant to her:

By health I mean the power to live a full, adult, living, breathing life in close contact with what I love ... I want to be all that I am capable of becoming ...

This statement reflects the idea that health is dynamic, that being healthy has something to do with achieving potential. It also implies that health represents a condition of mastery in which the extent of growth and the direction of potential lie with the individual. Many people share such a view. It is commonly claimed that the purpose of being healthy is to be able to live well, on one's own terms. In part, it implies the ability and opportunity to make decisions about one's own life. To decide on the meaning of health, then, is to make a value judgement.

Individuals define health on the basis of assumptions they make about the purpose and value of being healthy. Some assumptions which may be made about health are illustrated in Box 1.1. Clearly such a list could be extended considerably. Health has some elusive qualities that make it difficult to define. In addition, people have differing interpretations and aspirations. This creates a complex situation in which it is difficult to establish criteria to be considered in arriving at a definition of health. Is social conformity an important aspect of health? Can criminals be healthy people? Which is more important, emotional comfort or physical fitness? Some individuals appear to be obsessed with their health. Is this a healthy attitude? It is virtually impossible to achieve consensus on the answers to such questions, and to many more besides.

Professional statements about health are also value judgements, based on the goals and beliefs of the profession concerned. For instance, school teachers may tend to see the purpose of being healthy as related to being able to be socially useful. Such a view fits with the recent emphasis on citizenship in British school curricula; many teachers accept that a primary goal of the educational system is to prepare students for life in society. Similarly, health care professionals may assume that prevention of disease should command a prominent position in values related to health because they are convinced that absence of disease adds quality to life. This position could be seen to be reflected in the change in emphasis from ill health to health in the nursing curricula in the United Kingdom and other countries in recent years.

BOX 1.1	*Some assumptions about health.* Adapted from Health Education and the Nurse, National Nursing and Midwifery Consultative Committee, Scotland, 1983, published by the Scottish Home and Health Department

- Health means different things to different people.
- Health means more than the absence of disease or infirmity.
- Health implies adaptability.
- Optimum health varies.
- Health is necessary for the purposes of life and adds to the quality of life.

There is nothing wrong with either view. Indeed, it can be argued that the latter has traditionally been a proper professional perspective for nurses since the prevention of disease and care of the diseased person have justified nurses' professional existence. What is important is that health care professionals are aware of the origins and the limitations of their ideas about health, and that they are sensitive to the fact that individuals may want to decide for themselves about life and health. This perspective has become increasingly important with the many recent changes in the health care system and in the nature of nursing practice.

One way to guard against having a limited view of what it means to be healthy is to be open-minded in one's approach to people and to be aware that health is a matter of opinion and perception rather than of fact. It may be helpful to consider particular examples to bring this discussion into the context of reality. Take the case of a 19-year-old male who has survived a car crash but who is now paraplegic. Weeks of rehabilitation have enabled him to go home in the care of his parents. He manages most of his daily living activities and his feeling of responsibility prompts him to self-help in areas of skin and catheter care. He has talked about never achieving his former goal of driving a heavy goods vehicle and now is asking for career counselling about what he can do. Is this young man healthy? Or consider a 23-year-old former drug user who knows she is HIV-positive, though she does not presently have AIDS. She has been through a drug rehabilitation programme, and now works full-time in a project in her community which seeks to educate young people about drugs. Is she healthy?

The latter example also serves to suggest a way of approaching the notion of health which has gained popularity, the 'lifestyle' view of health. This, along with other views alluded to above, will be addressed in more detail later in this book.

In relation to the heading of this section, two things are obvious. First, a universally accepted definition of health is virtually impossible to find. Second, it is similarly impossible to predict the meaning that health will have for particular individuals. The exercise suggested in Activity 1.1 will help you to explore these ideas.

PLANNING FOR HEALTH

It is part of every nurse's responsibility to be involved in planning to maintain or improve the health of individuals or communities. Health is a dynamic concept; the health status of an individual may vary with time, place and circumstance. For working purposes, the nurse may consider 'health status' as a moveable point on a continuum. Figure 1.1 is a simple model of such a continuum. This model may be applied to communities as well as to individuals. An assumption that can be held about the model is that the extent and nature of ill health are neither predetermined nor a matter of chance and that it is possible to intervene to prevent or limit movement along the continuum in the direction of disease or disability and to facilitate movement towards optimal health. In other words, it is possible to plan for health.

Although optimal health and disease are at different ends of the continuum, it need not be assumed that there is a dichotomy of action between disease pre-

ACTIVITY 1.1

Consider the following quotations. To what extent do they seem to be referring to the same concept? To what extent do they agree with your 'meaning of health'?

■ 'Health is a state of complete physical, mental and social [and spiritual] well-being, and not merely the absence of disease or infirmity.' (World Health Organization 1947 [1988])

■ '[Health is] the extent to which an individual is able, on the one hand, to realize aspirations and satisfy needs and on the other hand, to change or cope with the environment ... a resource for everyday life, not the object of living ... a positive concept emphasizing social and personal resources as well as physical capacities.' (World Health Organization 1984)

■ '[Health is] freedom from illness, ability to function, fitness ... [A] "reserve" that can be diminished by self-neglect and accumulated by healthy behaviour ... largely determined by heredity, influenced by childhood and traumatic events.' (Blaxter 1990 p. 16)

■ 'Individuals may be considered healthy to the extent that they are capable of meeting the obligations and enjoying the rewards of living in their community.' (Smith & Jacobson 1988 p. 3)

■ Health is the 'ability of all people within the community to reach full mental, spiritual and physical potential by living in safety with vigor and purpose; meeting personal needs; meeting community responsibilities; adapting to change; and having trusting and caring relationships.' (Community Health Endowment of Lincoln 1998)

■ 'A health problem is the inability of the body to act on its master's will. Whatever that will may be. If one wishes to fly, then having no wings is a health problem according to that definition.' (Gideon TryAgain 2003)

vention and health promotion. Disease and health are interrelated and, in reality, what prevents disease promotes health and vice versa. This text assumes that disease prevention is an integral part of health promotion. It also assumes that health can be promoted and disease prevented not just for individuals who are currently disease-free but also for individuals with existing problems of ill health.

Influencing the patterns of health in given communities is achieved in a variety of ways, including environmental control, nutritional policy, immunization, screening and health education. Strategies for health promotion require the application of a range of fiscal, legal and social measures. Such strategies have to be widely based. The promotion of health is not the exclusive responsibility of health care professionals. Many agencies or entities are involved: education, employment, housing, transport and social services, as well as individuals themselves.

Three terms have been used traditionally in relation to strategies for the prevention of disease:

■ *Primary prevention*: action to prevent disease or disability before it occurs

■ *Secondary prevention*: action related to early detection and treatment of disease

■ *Tertiary prevention*: action to avoid needless progression or complications of disease.

FIGURE 1.1   *Continuum of health*

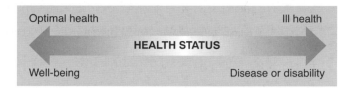

Examples of strategies for prevention

Examples of such strategies are given in Box 1.2. A comprehensive programme of prevention directed at any specific health problem may incorporate all three aspects. In drug-related programmes, for instance, primary prevention may be concerned with education and media campaigns which seek to influence mores and behaviour so that individuals choose to avoid the misuse of drugs. Secondary prevention attempts to identify drug users early, before addiction is

BOX 1.2   *Examples of strategies for prevention*

Primary prevention

- Immunization
- Provision of clean water
- Control of air pollution
- Fluoridation of water supplies
- Car seat belt legislation
- Teaching about healthy lifestyles (diet, exercise, safe sex, etc.)

Secondary prevention

- Eyesight screening in schools
- Deafness screening in certain occupations
- Breast self-examination and breast screening programmes
- Cervical screening
- Cholesterol screening
- Blood pressure screening

Tertiary prevention

- Teaching diet and insulin control in diabetes
- Controlling fits in epilepsy
- Limiting joint damage in rheumatic conditions
- Teaching about healthy lifestyle following myocardial infarction
- Teaching exercises following mastectomy
- Teaching skin care during and after radiotherapy.

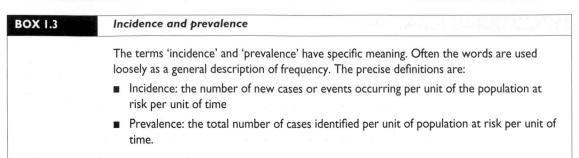

BOX 1.3 *Incidence and prevalence*

The terms 'incidence' and 'prevalence' have specific meaning. Often the words are used loosely as a general description of frequency. The precise definitions are:

■ Incidence: the number of new cases or events occurring per unit of the population at risk per unit of time

■ Prevalence: the total number of cases identified per unit of population at risk per unit of time.

established or damage is sustained. Tertiary prevention is directed at limiting the damaging effects of drug misuse, such as through drug rehabilitation and/or harm minimization programmes.

The nurse involved with health promotion strategies must have a rational basis for her plan; that is, as with any area of nursing practice, the nurse should base practice on the best available evidence. This means that as well as getting to know the particular individual or community, she must gather and interpret available health and vital statistics. The classic approach to health promotion employs the skills and insights of the epidemiologist.

Epidemiology is the study of the determinants of the incidence and the prevalence of disease (see Box 1.3). The epidemiologist collects data relating to the distribution and size of disease problems. By examining the data it is often possible to identify factors contributing to patterns of ill health. Nowadays, it is increasingly recognized that the epidemiological method may also be utilized to record patterns of health-related behaviour. As will be discussed later in this text, there is a danger in focusing too strongly on behaviour change as a 'cure' for society's health problems, but there is no doubt that behaviour does influence health.

Knowledge of the size of a disease problem and of the behavioural and other factors contributing to that problem allows for planning of services, both curative and preventive. The epidemiological approach to planning entails seeking answers to a series of questions such as:

■ Is there a problem?
■ How big is it?
■ How serious is it?
■ Who is affected by it?
■ What causes it?
■ Is it amenable to influence by educational methods or environmental engineering?
■ Will the costs of any such initiatives be justified by the outcomes that can be anticipated?

The following sections demonstrate some of the ways such questions are addressed and some ways of answering them.

MEASURING HEALTH

Health professionals are expected to demonstrate that their work is effective in improving health, and for this, measurements are needed. This applies to all aspects of their work, and it is particularly relevant, but also particularly problematic, for those activities that relate to health education and health promotion. If health can be described in a way which allows measurement, then it should be possible to assess the current state of health of either an individual or a community and to set goals for maintenance or improvement. This would also offer a means for gaining a 'before and after' view, making it possible to judge whether a given health intervention is being effective. Measurable goals thus allow for accurate evaluation.

Finding measurable aspects of a concept as elusive as health has proved difficult. Consider the World Health Organization's 1947 definition of health which was cited in Activity 1.1. It is impossible to demonstrate the achievement of such a goal. The difficulty is related to the problem of measurement. What is well-being? Exactly what does the individual have to feel or be able to do to be described as 'well'? Attempts have been made to distinguish levels of wellness and have been described (Galli 1978; Travis 2000). However, gaining agreement on the value to place on the various aspects considered to constitute wellness has proved, so far, an insurmountable task. A way of handling this problem has been to use negative indices of health, mainly in the form of mortality and morbidity statistics.

Mortality statistics

These are the records of deaths within a defined population. In Britain, births and deaths have had to be registered since 1836. The current requirements for recording them were laid down in the Births and Deaths Registration Act of 1953 for England and Wales, and in the Registration of Births, Deaths and Marriages (Scotland) Act 1965 and the Births and Deaths Registration (Northern Ireland) Order 1976 for the other two UK countries. When a death is registered, the cause of death is recorded along with the person's age, sex and social class. This means that figures from which to compile statistics relating to death rates from the various causes according to those basic variables are readily available. Moreover, since the records have been kept for many decades, it is possible to study trends in the pattern of diseases.

Morbidity statistics

These record the amount of illness in a community. There are many parameters, such as general practitioner consultations, sickness absence, hospital admission and reports of illness surveys. Morbidity data are less readily available at national level than are mortality figures. Survey data about illness are often generated within research projects which look specifically at one disease or group of diseases, or at specific segments of the population, and since researchers have different purposes for their data, they tend to record them differently. Consequently the available picture is somewhat patchy. A regular source of information in the UK is provided by the General Household Survey

(GHS) which is conducted annually with a sample size of 30,000 persons. This multipurpose household survey has been carried out since 1971, except for breaks in 1997-98 and 1999-2000. At the time of writing, the most recent year reported is 2000-01 and is available online from the UK Data Archive. The health section of the survey collects data on general practitioner consultations, outpatient visits and acute and long-standing illness. The data depend, of course, upon the self-reports of the people interviewed, and are subject therefore to the vagaries of perception and memory. This makes them difficult to interpret. Other sources of morbidity data include figures relating to sickness absence and hospitalisation, and national surveys of general practice consultations. For example, the Office of Population Censuses and Surveys (OPCS) reported the 4th National Study of Morbidity Statistics from General Practice for 1991/92 for the UK (McCormick et al 1995), and ISD Scotland reported a survey of the 'Top 5 Most Common Reasons for Consulting a GP' by sex and age group for the year ending December 2000.

A comprehensive account of sources of mortality and morbidity statistics is given in the Central Statistical Office's *Guide to Official Statistics*, most recently published in 2000 and available online as well as in 'hard copy'.

In countries such as the UK, Canada, and Australia, the availability of reasonably accurate morbidity and mortality statistics allows the determination of the extent of disease problems in given populations. They can also be utilized to help establish the seriousness of any problem and the scope for prevention. This is a much greater challenge in some other countries, such as those of southern Africa, where such statistics are difficult to collect or locate, while there are serious disease problems that need tackling.

Population statistics

To make sense of data relating to health, it is necessary to have some background information about the size of the population under study and its composition with regard to factors such as age, sex and social class. The main sources of such information in Britain today are data gathered during the Census which is carried out at 10-yearly intervals. This began in 1801 and was missed only once, in 1941, during the Second World War. The Census provides information on numbers of persons, their age, sex, occupation, nationality, ethnic group, residence and type of housing. Questions covering certain additional topics are sometimes included. The Office for National Statistics (ONS) (formerly the Office of Population Censuses and Surveys) for England and Wales, the General Register Office for Scotland (GROS), and the General Register Office for Northern Ireland (GRO-NI) are the Government agencies responsible for arranging the Census and analysing the data. Further statistics are provided from data gathered from the registration of births, mentioned earlier, as well as marriages, deaths, divorces and adoptions, which are also required by law to be registered.

Epidemiologists gather data from the Census and the various registrations to draw up a profile of population characteristics and trends. Health-related statistics, such as morbidity, mortality and use of services figures, are collected in order to determine the frequency of a disease or an ill-health problem or health-related behaviour, and are often expressed as rates rather than as crude figures. Using rates helps to indicate the size of a problem. Clearly it is not

TABLE 1.1	Common rates used in assessing the health status of populations		
Name of rate	**Event counted**	**Population at risk**	
Crude death rate	Deaths	Total population	
Birth rate	Births	Total population	
Fertility rate	Births	Females 15-44/49	
Stillbirth rate	Stillbirths	Total births (live and still)	
Infant mortality	Deaths under 1 year	Live births	
Neonatal mortality	Deaths under 1 month	Live births	
Perinatal mortality	Deaths under 1 week and stillbirths	Total births (live and still)	

much use to be able to say that 100 people have died of a certain disease. That reveals nothing about the size and seriousness of the problem. It doesn't place the 100 people in any context – that is, 100 people out of how many? In what type of population? Over what period of time?

Using rates helps to avoid these difficulties, because a rate refers to the number of events recorded in relation to the population at risk over a specified period of time. There are three types of rates: crude rates, adjusted (or standardized) rates and specific rates. Crude rates are expressed in terms of a total population. There are limitations to this, as not all members of the population share the same risks. A man, for example, is at no risk of cervical cancer, while a woman is at no risk of testicular cancer. To avoid these limitations, adjusted or specific rates are used. Table 1.1 shows some rates which are commonly referred to in assessing the health status of different populations.

In some ways, examination of the mortality statistics gives the most accurate picture of the pattern of disease in a community. Some distortions of these rates do occur due to difficulties in diagnosis, changes in disease classification, or selective avoidance of diagnosis by doctors, but it is generally agreed that the cause of death recorded at present in the UK and other westernized societies is reliable. However, a limitation of mortality statistics is that they give no idea of the nature of the ill-health problem nor of its impact on society. Certain health conditions that are of interest may not appear as such in mortality statistics if they themselves are not the direct cause of death. This can occur with AIDS, for example, which may not be given as the cause of death; the specific condition from which the person with AIDS dies may be recorded on its own as the cause of death. Morbidity statistics, on the other hand, allow us to consider the amount of ill health which exists and to estimate its social and treatment costs.

As mortality and morbidity statistics are negative indices of health, that is, they indicate ill health, it must be remembered that to assess the health of a community solely on the basis of such information is to miss something of the essence of health. Nevertheless, they constitute probably the best source of reliable information currently available on which to base plans for health. The prevention of disease is not the last word in health promotion, but it can be argued that it provides a necessary first step.

CURRENT ILL HEALTH IN BRITAIN

Mortality

Historical comparisons

The pattern of ill health in Britain has changed drastically during the last century or more. A rough-and-ready measure of this is the crude death rate, which for England and Wales was 21.4 per thousand population in the period 1841-1845, 12.0 per thousand in 1931-1935 (OPCS 1992), and only 10.5 per thousand for 1996-2000 (ONS 2002). The infant mortality rate has fallen even more rapidly. For the period 1841-1845, there were 148 infant deaths per thousand live births, whereas in 1931-1935 there were 62, and by 1996-2000 just 6.

Most people, therefore, are now living longer. For example, in England and Wales in 1841 a new baby could expect to live 40.2 years if it was a boy, or 42.2 years if it was a girl. By 1901, these life expectancy rates had risen to 48.5 and 52.4 respectively, and by 1950 to 66.4 and 71.5. Calculations for 2001 indicate that in the UK a baby boy's life expectancy was 75.13 years and a baby girl's was 80.66 years (CIA 2001). Thus within 160 years, life expectancy has increased nearly 87% for males and just over 91% for females (see Figure 1.2).

In the 19th century the main causes of mortality, once the hazards of birth were surmounted, were infectious diseases such as scarlet fever, measles, whooping cough, diphtheria, typhoid fever, cholera, tuberculosis and small-pox. In the 100 years from 1875 till the mid-1970s, death rates from these diseases had been reduced by 99%. Since the 1950s there have been dramatic falls in the incidence of infectious diseases. Diphtheria and acute poliomyelitis have been virtually eradicated, and tuberculosis, though still present, no longer

FIGURE 1.2   *Life expectancy at birth in England and Wales*

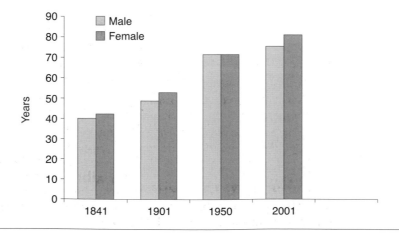

makes an important contribution to mortality rates in Britain. Some infectious diseases still occur from time to time; for example, 1978 brought the worst epidemic of whooping cough since 1957, and there are periodic small epidemics of various strains of influenza. However, the major threats to life in the UK in recent times have been chronic degenerative diseases rather than acute infections (DHSS 1976; Statistics Division, Department of Health 2002).

The current main causes of death in Britain are diseases of the circulatory system (especially ischaemic heart disease), cancer, and cerebrovascular disease (especially stroke), in that order. Other major causes include diseases of the respiratory, central nervous, and digestive systems, as well as injury and poisoning (OPCS 1993, 1994; Statistics Division, Department of Health 2002). However, these statistics are very general, and there are interesting differences in the rates of death from specific causes according to age, sex and geographical area.

Mortality by age group and gender

According to UK mortality statistics for the year 1999 (WHO 2003), most deaths during the first year of life (excluding the first month) were attributed to 'signs, symptoms and ill-defined conditions', the majority of these being Sudden Infant Death Syndrome (SIDS). Apart from specifically birth-related problems, other causes of death before the age of 1 year included congenital anomalies, infections, diseases of the nervous and respiratory systems, and accidents. Between the ages of 1 and 34 years, deaths are few, and many are due to accidents rather than to disease, with road traffic accidents being a particular problem. Accidental injury is the most frequent cause of death in both males and females in the groups for ages 1 to 4 years and 15 to 24 years, and among males in the 5-14 group and the 25-34 group. For females ages 5-14 and 25-34, malignant neoplasms constitute a more common cause of death, with accidents being second. Malignant neoplasms rank second for males in the 5-14 group, but not in the 15-24 or 25-34 groups, in which suicide becomes the second most common cause of death. This is despite there being greater numbers of deaths from neoplastic disease among males than among females in the 15-24 group, which illustrates the relative significance of suicide as a cause of death among males in these age groups – the numbers are not high in absolute terms, but they are high relative to other causes of death in these groups in which deaths are relatively few.

Between the ages of 35 and 44, neoplasms increase as a cause of death, becoming the most common cause among women and second most common among men, with diseases of the circulatory system becoming the most common cause of death for men and second for women. This pattern continues from ages 45 through 74. Ischaemic heart disease is responsible for the greatest proportion of cardiac deaths. Within the broad category of neoplastic disease, breast cancer increases as a cause of death among women, while cancer of the respiratory system accounts for an increasing proportion of deaths among men. Among both sexes, cancer of the digestive organs becomes increasingly evident. In the 65-74 age group, the number of deaths from disease of the circulatory system among women has pulled almost level with deaths from malignant neoplasms. A noticeable rate of death from cerebrovascular disease begins to appear in this age range (WHO 2003).

| FIGURE 1.3 | *Major causes of death by age group* |

Age group	Major causes of death (in rank order)		
<1 year	Sudden infant death syndrome, congenital anomalies, infectious diseases, diseases of nervous and respiratory systems, accidents		
1-4 years	Accidental injury		
5-14 years	M–Accidental injury, malignant neoplasms		
	F–Malignant neoplasms, accidental injury		
15-24 years	Accidental injury	M–Suicide	
		F–Malignant neoplasms	
25-34 years	M–Accidental injury, suicide		
	F–Malignant neoplasms, accidental injury		
35-44 years	M–Diseases of circulatory system, neoplasms		
	F–Neoplasms, diseases of the circulatory system		
45-74 years	Diseases of circulatory system (esp. ischaemic heart disease)	M–Cancer of respiratory system, cancer of digestive organs	
		F–Breast cancer, cancer of digestive organs	
75+ years	Diseases of circulatory system (esp. IHD, cerebrovascular & arterial disease), cancer (digestive & respiratory systems; female breast; genitourinary, esp. prostate; pneumonia; chronic obstructive airways disease; diseases of central nervous system; diseases of endocrine system (esp. diabetes mellitus)		
ALL AGES	**Diseases of the circulatory system, malignant neoplasms, pneumonia, cerebrovascular disease**		

Among people aged 75 and beyond, many of the major causes of death remain proportionately similar to the previous decade, but the numbers rise, as would be expected. The greatest number of deaths are accounted for by circulatory disease, particularly ischaemic heart disease, cerebrovascular disease and arterial disease. Cancer continues to be the second largest major category of causes of death, most noticeably of the digestive system, respiratory system, female breast, and genitourinary system, especially the prostate in men. Other respiratory diseases, including pneumonia and chronic obstructive airways disease, also contribute. Other diseases which appear as frequent causes of death for the first time include diseases of the central nervous system and the endocrine system, especially diabetes mellitus (WHO 2003) (see Figure 1.3).

Taking all ages together, the four most common causes of death are diseases of the circulatory system, malignant neoplasms, pneumonia and cerebrovascular disease. This illustrates an interesting point: while pneumonia never appears as a top cause of death in any age group, in overall terms it figures importantly. This is because it is responsible for a meaningful, though never huge, number of deaths in virtually all age groups. In looking at Figure 1.3, the reader should keep in mind that the numbers of deaths are very small in the younger age groups.

It can be seen in the information discussed above that differences exist between male and female mortality rates. In fact, male mortality rates exceed female mortality rates at every stage in the life span until age 75 (WHO 2003), and this has been true since records were first kept. The net result is a preponderance of females in the elderly population.

Mortality by geographical area and social class

Statistics also show that some groups in the population are likely to live longer than others. There are regional variations in age-specific mortality rates; for example, in the UK someone living in the southeast of England in 1980 had a better chance of reaching retirement age than someone living in Wales or the North (DHSS 1980). This is a fairly recent phenomenon: in the 19th century the southeast of England recorded high death rates, while the far north was a much healthier place to live. Mortality statistics from 2000 demonstrate an interesting pattern among the countries of the UK. General death rates (rates including all age groups, from all causes) are highest for men in Scotland and lowest for men in Northern Ireland, and highest for women in Wales and lowest in Northern Ireland (ONS 2002). For the major categories of cause of death, Scotland and Wales tend to share the top positions, with England in third place and Northern Ireland in fourth place.

As well as regional variations in mortality, there are differences related to social class. For the purposes of analysing health statistics, the most frequently applied categorization of social class is the one used by the Registrar General. This categorizes people according to occupation. The classification used since 1970 is shown in Box 1.4.

A study of inequalities in health in Britain was commissioned by the Department of Health and Social Security (DHSS) in 1977, and this resulted in a landmark report, the Black Report, which was published three years later (DHSS 1980). The study revealed that in the Britain of the 1970s, a child born to parents in Class I, provided he did not change his class, was likely to live five years longer than a child born to parents in Class V. Class differences in mortality were found to persist throughout the human life span, with mortality tending to rise with falling status. The babies and children of unskilled manual workers were less likely to survive their first year than those of professionals. Twice as many babies of Class V died within the first month, and between 1 and 12 months four times as many girls and five times as many boys died. The risk of death from fire, falls or drowning between 1 and 14 years was ten times higher for boys in Class V than in Class I.

Class differences in mortality were less marked for adults, but a class gradient in favour of the upper classes could be demonstrated for many, though by no means all, causes of death. Class was significant for both sexes in infectious and parasitic diseases, blood diseases and diseases of the respiratory and genitourinary systems. There were steep class gradients for women in circulatory disease

BOX 1.4	Class occupational category, with percentage of total population	
I	Professional (e.g. accountant, doctor, lawyer)	5%
II	Intermediate (e.g. manager, school teacher, nurse)	18%
IIIn	Skilled non-manual (e.g. clerical worker, secretary, shop assistant)	12%
IIIm	Skilled manual (e.g. bus driver, butcher, coal-face worker, carpenter)	38%
IV	Partly skilled (e.g. agricultural worker, bus conductor, postman)	18%
V	Unskilled (e.g. labourer, cleaner, dock worker)	9%

and in endocrine, nutritional and metabolic diseases and for men in malignant neoplasms, accidents and diseases of the nervous system (DHSS 1980).

A follow-up study to the Black Report was carried out during the 1980s (Whitehead 1987). It revealed that, disappointingly, 'serious social inequalities in health' persisted. People in the lower social classes retained higher death rates than those higher up, and this applied at every stage of life from birth through old age. The study found evidence that unemployment had a direct negative effect on health, and striking regional disparities remained. It demonstrated, in brief, that not only had inequalities in health in Britain persisted, the gap had continued to widen.

Another study carried out during the same period looked at the issue of inequalities in health from a particular perspective relevant to health education and health promotion (Blaxter 1990). This study found that positive health behaviours or 'lifestyles' did not result in equally positive effects on health in the different social classes. At the upper end of the social scale, a healthy change in lifestyle led to the achievement of a significant health gain, while at the lower end of the scale a similar change in lifestyle resulted in only a minimal health gain. One conclusion that could be drawn from this is that differences in healthiness of lifestyle between the different social classes is not a sufficient explanation for the inequalities in health.

Occupation, as categorized by the Registrar General, provides a very crude tool with which to judge social class, and one which may need refining. Income, property, education and housing tenure have been proposed as alternative variables which might be used to stratify the population (DHSS 1980). However, the scheme based on occupation continues to be the most commonly used. Minor changes are made regularly, such as the moving of an occupation from one class to another, and the scheme was renamed from the Registrar General's Social Classes (RGSC) to Social Class Based on Occupation in 1990 (Rose 1995). Nonetheless, even the crude tool based on occupation generates such consistent results that there can be little doubt that real inequalities of health persist in Britain, at least on the basis of existing mortality statistics.

More recent British studies (Green 1994; Noble et al 1994; Mitchell et al 2000) have demonstrated that the gap between poverty and wealth continues to enlarge, so it seems reasonable to suppose that the health gap is similarly continuing to increase.

Morbidity

The available morbidity statistics provide further interesting information about the state of Britain's health. Cardiovascular disease and cancer may be the greatest killer diseases of modern times, but dental caries is probably the most prevalent disease, especially in Scotland, though there has been some improvement within the past two decades. A study carried out in 1983 showed that 70% of Scottish 9-year-olds and 48% of English 9-year-olds had some decay in their permanent teeth, and Scottish 15-year-olds had known decay in an average of 8.4 teeth compared with 5.6 teeth and 6.7 teeth in their English and Welsh counterparts, respectively (OPCS 1983). In 1988, 33% of Scottish adults aged 45 to 54 had had all their teeth extracted, compared with 15% of English adults of the same ages (Scottish Office Home and Health Department 1991). This represented an improvement from 54% and 28% respectively in

| FIGURE 1.4 | *Full dental extractions among adults aged 45-54 in England and Scotland* |

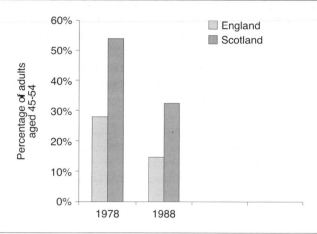

1978, but still represented a far from satisfactory state of dental health (see Figure 1.4). Government reports from 1998 and 1999 showed that although Scotland's dental health was improving, it was not on track to meet targets set in 1991 for the year 2000, and the date for meeting these targets was revised to 2005 (SODH 1998; NHS Scotland 1999). The British diet is notably high in sugar content, especially in Scotland, and problems have been found to be particularly marked in disadvantaged areas, with 60% of 3-year-olds being reported to have dental caries in 1998 (SODH 1998).

Morbidity statistics from general practice reveal that the most common reasons for consulting a doctor in Britain are related to respiratory disease. In

| TABLE 1.2 | *Reasons for consultations (specific), England and Wales, 1991/92* |

Rates per 10,000 person years at risk*

Reason	Rate
Acute upper respiratory infections of multiple or unspecified site	772
Acute bronchitis and bronchitis	719
Asthma	425
Disorders of conjuctiva	415
Essential hypertension	412
Disorders of external ear	409
Acute pharyngitis	409
Acute tonsillitis	407
Ill-defined intestinal infections	394
Other and unspecified disorders of back	372

* As the statistics are based on each patient being registered with a practice for a full year, figures have to be adjusted to take into account those who were not registered for a full year. For example if one patient is registered for eight months and another for four months, they would be counted as one person year.

ACTIVITY 1.2

Look at Table 1.3, which displays statistical information for Scotland for the year 2000 regarding the 'Top 5 Most Common Reasons for Consulting a GP'. While examining the table, you should keep a few points in mind:

1. If a certain 'reason for consulting' does not appear in the table at any particular point, that does not mean it does not exist at all for that age group or sex. It just means that it didn't rank among the 'Top 5' at that point.

2. The naming of complaints or reasons for attending is not an exact science, so sometimes such data cannot be treated as foolproof. For example, an asthmatic may attend the GP with an upper respiratory infection (URI), and the reason for the consultation might then be listed as either asthma or as a URI; or a woman who is menopausal may attend with depression and anxiety, so there are three possible ways of listing her reason for attending.

3. Not all reasons for consulting relate to existing illness complaints. Examples would be child health surveillance and family planning.

In looking at the data displayed in the table, what patterns do you see? Can you think of some possible explanations for these patterns?

TABLE 1.3   *Top 5 most common reasons for consulting a general practitioner by sex and age group, for year ending December 2000.* From ISD Scotland National Statistics

Reason for consulting a General practitioner	Under 5		5-14		15-24		25-44		45-64		65-74		75-84		85+		All ages	
	M	F	M	F	M	F	M	F	M	F	M	F	M	F	M	F	M	F
Resp. infections (upper/lower tract)	1/5	1	1	1	5	5	5		4		2	2	2	2	1	2	2	2/5
Child health surveillance & vaccination	2	2/5																
Otitis media	3	3	4	5														
Eczema/dermatitis	4	4		4														
Sore throat			2	2	2	4												
Asthma			3															
Verruca/wart			5	3														
Drug abuse					1		3											
Family planning – misc						1		4										
Oral contraceptive						2		5										
Acne					3													
Depression						3	2	1	3	2	4						4	1
Trauma – misc					4													
Back problems							1	3	2	4	3			4			3	4
Anxiety							4	2	5	5								5
Hypertension									1	3	1	1	1	1	4	1	1	2
Menopause										1								
Coronary heart disease											3		5					
Chronic obstructive airways dis											4		3		3			
Diabetes											5							
Osteoarthritis												5		3				
Heart failure													4		2	5		
Urinary tract infection														5				3
General – misc															5	4		
Dementia																3		

England and Wales, for example, respiratory illness accounted for 31% of all GP consultations in 1991/92 (OPCS 1995). In Scotland in 2000, respiratory illness ranked among the top five reasons for GP consultations among both sexes in all age groups except women in the 24-44 and 45-64 age groups (ISD Scotland 2001). Other common complaints can be seen in Table 1.2 which shows the top ranking presenting complaints in England in Wales for 1991/92.

SOME INTERNATIONAL COMPARISONS

The above discussion has focused primarily on the UK. Readers from other countries may be aware of similarities and/or differences in the health and ill-health profiles of their countries. It is interesting to consider what some of these similarities and differences are.

The health picture in different countries can be explored by looking at statistics that relate to life, illness and death. Consider the information in Table 1.4, for example. It shows the infant mortality rate (IMR), which is the number of deaths of children under one year old per 1000 live births, the maternal mortality rate (MMR), which is the number of maternal deaths per 100,000 live births, and the average life expectancy at birth, for a range of countries. It should be kept in mind that not all these statistics are entirely accurate, or necessarily exactly comparable, because such data may be collected and counted in different ways in different countries. However, they have been compiled by experts in population studies and are sufficient to provide a general picture of the situation in the various countries.

Another way of exploring the health picture in different countries is to look at the leading causes of death. Box 1.5 shows the five leading causes of death in three countries. Note the similarities between Canada and Australia, and note how the list for South Africa differs from the other two. An obvious problem with such classifications is that they can only represent a limited view of the causes. For example, when 'cancer' or 'neoplasm' is listed, this will include a wide variation in types of cancer. Similarly, 'infectious diseases' covers a wide range of specific infections. Looked at from another perspective, there are some conditions that may not appear in the list but may nevertheless be important causative factors. An example would be HIV/AIDS, which is

BOX 1.5	Five leading causes of death in three countries	
Australia (Australian Bureau of Statistics 2002)	**Canada** (Health Canada/Santé Canada 2000)	**South Africa** (Statistics South Africa 2002)
Cancer	Diseases of the circulatory system	Infectious and parasitic diseases
Ischaemic heart disease	Cancer	External causes (in males only)
Stroke	Respiratory diseases	Diseases of the circulatory system
Chronic lower respiratory disease	Unintentional injuries	Ill-defined causes
Accidents	Diseases of the digestive system	Diseases of the respiratory system
		Neoplasms (in females only)

TABLE 1.4   *Some international health data comparisons – 2002/2003.* PRB 2002, 2003

Country	Infant mortality rate	Maternal mortality rate	Life expectancy at birth Male	Female
Albania	12	31	72	76
Australia	5.1	6	77	82
Bangladesh	66	600	59	59
Brazil	33	260	65	73
Canada	5.3	6	77	82
China	32	60	69	73
Denmark	4.9	15	75	79
Estonia	9	80	65	76
Ethiopia	107	1800	41	43
France	4.2	20	76	83
Germany	4.3	12	75	81
Greece	5.9	2	76	81
Hungary	7.2	23	68	76
India	66	440	62	64
Iraq	103	370	56	59
Israel	5.3	8	77	81
Jamaica	24	120	73	77
Japan	3.0	12	78	85
Jordan	22	41	69	71
Malta	3.4	0[a]	74	80
Mexico	25	65	73	78
Netherlands	5.4	10	76	81
New Zealand	5.3	15	76	81
Nigeria	75	1100	52	52
Palestinian Territory	26	-[b]	71	74
Philippines	26	240	67	72
Russia	15	75	59	72
South Africa	57	340	53	54
United Kingdom	5.4	10	75	80
United States of America	6.9	12	74	80
World	54	400	65	69

[a] *This figure must be viewed in light of the country's small population. There were no maternal deaths in childbirth in this particular year, but that does not mean there is never such a death in Malta.*

[b] *Figure not available.*

ACTIVITY 1.3

Consider the data displayed in Table 1.4 and Box 1.5. What do you notice that is interesting, puzzling, or perhaps shocking? You might, for example, look at the differences between data about males and females. Can you think of any possible explanations for the differences? You will notice that there are large differences in infant and maternal mortality rates in different countries. Can you see any patterns in these differences? Again, can you think of possible explanations for the differences?

often not listed as cause of death. Instead, the specific condition that actually precipitated the death is listed, but that condition may be a consequence of the HIV/AIDS. Thus the enormous differences in HIV/AIDS rates between different countries, such as the countries of Africa as compared with western Europe or North America, would not be evident in lists of causes of death.

Table 1.4 and Box 1.5 touch on just some of the types of data that are available about health and ill health. There are many web sources of such data, and you might like to try to find some for yourself on topics or countries that interest you. If you need guidance on how to go about doing this, members of your academic or library staff will be able to offer advice.

POSITIVE VIEWS OF HEALTH

It is noticeable that in the previous sections, the discussion related to health has focused largely on aspects of its absence, that is, on evidence of ill health. There is an obvious reason for this: it is easier to identify elements of ill health, and to find ways to measure these, than it is to find ways of measuring positive health, especially since health means such different things to different people. Various attempts have been made to do this, however. One commonly used instrument is the General Health Questionnaire (GHQ) (Goldberg & Williams 1988; McDowell & Newell 1996). This questionnaire is widely used for a broad range of studies in which a measure of health or quality of life is sought, and it has been adapted for use in many languages and cultures. It is also flexible in that it has variations containing as few as 12 items and as many as 60 items. Thus its use can be tailored to the needs of a variety of studies. However, although the GHQ includes many items that ask positive questions about health, such as, 'Have you recently felt that you are playing a useful part in things?', it also includes many items that touch on ill health, such as, 'Have you recently been feeling run down and out of sorts?' So again, the individual's level of health is being judged, at least in part, by the presence of ill health, though not by the identification of specific diseases.

The reader may have noticed that there is a clear difference between using something like the GHQ and using mortality and morbidity data to measure health. The GHQ asks individuals about their perception of their own health, so it looks at health from a subjective viewpoint rather than identifying and counting up examples of poor health. This could be seen as a good thing, if we are looking for evidence of health rather than illness, because it allows individuals to judge their health on their own terms. However, it does not take us any further in the search for objective ways to measure positive instances of health in a population. That is, we still don't know what we could 'count' that would tell us the state of people's health (rather than ill health).

One further thing we might do is to look at data on the actions people take to preserve their health or to identify health problems early. This might include, for example, looking at the rates of attendance for dental or eye checkups, or the take-up rates for breast or cervical screening, or the immunization rates for preventable infectious diseases such as measles, mumps and rubella. Such information may indeed be useful in the planning of health promotion or education programmes. But once again they tend to focus on conditions of ill health, albeit in their prevention, so it is an 'absence of disease' view of health that is at work, rather than a view of what health itself consists of in positive terms. Thus this thorny issue remains difficult to resolve, and we must move on as best we can within the limits of what it is possible to do.

HEALTH EDUCATION AND HEALTH PROMOTION

Examination of current ill health in society reveals quite clearly that many of today's problems could be prevented. Some diseases have their origins in the behaviour of individuals, in the things they eat or the lifestyle patterns they choose. Other factors governing ill health are not within the individual's control but are deeply embedded in the value system, organizations and structures of society. Consider the information offered in Activity 1.2 in relation to these personal and contextual factors affecting the health of individuals.

The responsibility for any person's health lies strongly, but certainly not only, with that individual. There are also collective and expert responsibilities. The present dominance of preventable diseases demands intervention. In this, nurses have a part to play. They have the same individual and collective responsibilities as other members of society. In addition, they have the expert's responsibility to promote positive health, such as by helping others become aware of health-related issues and responsibilities. That is where health promotion and the nurse's role unite.

ACTIVITY 1.4

■ Data for Scotland show that in recent years all-sites cancer rates (i.e. rates that include cancer in any part of the body) have remained relatively steady in both males and females, but from 1930-32 to 1970-72 the rates from cancer of the trachea, bronchus and lung rose steeply for males and females in most age groups. Male rates were much higher than female rates, but since 1970-72 the male rates have shown more improvement than female rates. These rates can be seen to fit logically with smoking habits during those periods. How might these facts be related to individual behaviour, social values and societal structures?

■ Between 1982 and 1992 rates of death from road transport accidents dropped in Scotland by 37%. Compulsory seat belt legislation was introduced in February 1983 (Registrar General Scotland 1983). What issues are suggested by the apparent relationship between these two facts?

Earlier in this chapter, health was presented as a moveable point on a continuum. The health status of individuals or of communities may be influenced by planned strategies directed at health promotion. One of the main ways of influencing the health of a community is health education, which is a planned process aimed at helping individuals and communities achieve and maintain a level of health which is appropriate for them. Many different types of activity are labelled 'health education'. For this reason the term may be considered as an umbrella which encompasses a number of communication activities concerned with promoting the health of both the well and the sick.

Some of the main types of health education activities are:

- community health education programmes directed by health education officers
- health promotion through the public media
- education of patients or clients, conducted by health professionals
- school health education programmes, carried out by teachers
- self-help activities enabled by voluntary groups, community workers or health care professionals.

Generally speaking, the purpose is to promote health. Since health means different things to different people, there are many definitions of health education, and a wide range of goals. Levin (1977) summarized the following goals:

1. contribute to self-fulfilment of individuals and promote their well-being as individuals;
2. enhance the ability of people to cope effectively with health promotion, health maintenance and illness control;
3. reduce undesired risks of disease and illness;
4. help people maintain personal and civil integrity while receiving health care; and
5. create more active individual and community participation in the health system by increasing, (a) personal competence in self-care, and (b) social skills in working within the formal health system (p. 632).

One might add to this a concomitant political or utilitarian goal, namely to reduce or limit the drain on the public purse created by ill health which could be prevented by changes in the behaviour of individuals.

More recently, Ewles and Simnet (1995) have listed the aims of health promotion as being to raise health awareness, to change attitudes and behaviour, to improve knowledge, to empower individuals and to bring about societal and environmental change. In the USA, national goals of health promotion have been stated within a campaign called 'Healthy People 2010', launched by the Office of Disease Prevention and Health Promotion to improve the nation's health. These goals are: to help individuals of all ages increase life expectancy *and* improve their quality of life, and to eliminate health disparities among different segments of the population (US Department of Health and Human Services 2000).

Although these various sets of goals or aims are differently worded, many similarities are inherent in their elements. These are relevant to the work of nurses in a wide range of roles, and a key aspect of health promotion that nurses are regularly involved with is health education.

Nurses are involved as health educators both in the hospital and in the community, and their activities in this respect relate to all points on the continuum of health (refer to Figure 1.1). Community education is channelled to the 'healthy' population: those who feel well, who have neither symptoms nor clinical signs of disease. It takes many forms. Examples might be: teaching school children about brushing their teeth; running antenatal classes for prospective parents; conducting teenage group discussions about relationships and 'safe sex'; teaching breast self-examination to women in a well-woman clinic.

Patient education is intended for the person undergoing diagnosis, treatment or rehabilitation. Examples are: lessons on stoma management to a person with a colostomy; instruction on insulin injection to a person with diabetes; explanation to a person scheduled for surgery about what to expect in the anaesthetic room; pre-discharge discussion with a person with angina about lifestyle factors related to ischaemic heart disease.

Whatever the goals, it is basic to all health education, first, that personal or collective behaviour influences health status and, second, that it is possible to change the health-related behaviour of individuals or communities by planned purposeful activity. The concept of planned influence may appear to be at variance with the goal of helping people maintain personal and civil integrity. Problems do arise in practice and are resolved according to the ideological and ethical position of the individual health educator.

ETHICAL ISSUES IN HEALTH PROMOTION

Since the definition of health depends upon value judgement, there are bound to be ethical issues related to health promotion. These present a number of challenges to health professionals.

It is widely accepted that every individual has the right to assume responsibility for his own health, to define it for himself and to live accordingly. The problem is that to live to the full is not always to survive best. Many ill-health problems of today are related to lifestyle choices which favour the development of chronic degenerative diseases. When people consciously choose what to do about health they often disregard the evidence of risks involved in behaviours such as cigarette smoking, eating a high-fat diet, indulging in casual sexual activity, and drinking and driving. Such behaviour can result in conditions which not only damage the health of the individual but also are costly in social and economic terms.

Occasionally people act in ways that are counter to good health because they do not know any better. However, that is becoming increasingly rare in westernized society as information sources expand with expanding technology. Usually the facts are available, but they may be ignored. One possible reason for this may be that the person concerned does not value wellness or the avoidance of disease. The tantalizing aroma emanating from a fish and chip shop may offer the prospect of short-term gratification which outweighs the long-term concern for healthy arteries in later life. Watching sport on television may provide a more enticing source of enjoyment than playing tennis or swimming, despite the potential reward of greater cardiovascular fitness and a more supple old age offered by such activities. Enjoyment of the present has an immediately understandable meaning, while possible implications for a distant future may seem vague and uncertain, and can easily be ignored. Added to this is the fact that different individual views on what constitutes health or wellness mean that not everyone accepts the definitions assumed by health professionals. For example, some people might feel that the relaxation they gain from smoking represents greater wellness to them than the wellness they would presumably achieve by giving it up. Or a mother might feel that serving her husband and children the chips they demand leads to a degree of family harmony at meal times that gives her a greater level of wellness than would be gained by serving healthier food amidst family discord. However well such people understand the health information presented to them, their view of what wellness means to them is likely to have a strong influence on their behaviour.

Another reason for not responding to readily available information is that people do not necessarily make conscious choices about health-related behaviour. Habits may be acquired over the years as part of a person's socialization. Some people slip into regular heavy drinking of alcohol because they have grown up seeing this behaviour in their role models: a night out with friends from college or work means a night out drinking; drinking appears sophisticated or manly, according to a person's social identification, in images on television and in the cinema; peer pressure to 'stand one's round', and to accept one's share of everyone else's round, is too strong to resist. People may choose to spend their weekends hill-walking, going to the races, sailing, watching television, visiting antique shops, or any of various other leisure pursuits, for exactly the same reason – it is what they have grown up with and see as normal or accepted, or it is done by the people they admire or want to share activities with. Some lifestyles are virtually absorbed rather than chosen, and if a conscious choice is made, it may not be made on rational grounds.

Influencing the health status of individuals engaged in unhealthy behaviour may require planned purposeful intervention, and that in turn may involve an element of persuasion. This presents a dilemma. The rights of the individual may be at odds with the needs of society, or with the individual's needs as seen by the agents of society. Health professionals have to resolve the issues implied by this dilemma in order to be involved in health promotion and to reduce the personal, social and economic costs of illness and premature death.

One question that arises is the extent to which it is reasonable to limit personal freedom in order to improve the quality of health of a community. There is no easy answer to such a question. In exploring the issue it should be recognized that there is no such thing as absolute freedom. With any degree of freedom comes the responsibility of considering the effects of that freedom on others. It is not unknown for personal freedom to be sacrificed to the common good, as with legislation to control road traffic, or to regulate antisocial noise in residential areas.

Health educators are often asked to decide whether it is ethical to attempt to influence the choice of others. Some would argue that it is unethical not to. There is, after all, no values vacuum; there are many persuasive agencies at work in a free society. Many of these offer anti-health messages, the tobacco industry and some alcohol producers being examples. Moreover, the expenditure available for such advertising campaigns usually swamps the relatively small sums available for health promotion.

It can also be argued in favour of health education that individuals have a right to know what will affect their health, even if they are going to choose not to act upon it. The persuasion issue can thus be avoided by assuming that all the health educator needs to do is present the facts about health without bias. But can bias be avoided? In itself, the decision to attempt to prevent disease introduces bias. Achieving a value-free presentation of facts may be more difficult than it first appears. And what of individuals who declare that they want to live free from worry, and who consider that they have a right *not to know* what is harmful to their health? Some of the ways in which health educators respond to these ethical issues are addressed in Chapter 2, and the topic of ethics is revisited in Chapter 11.

REFERENCES

Abu Reidah MA-H 2003 Physical and Psychological Health in Islam. Faculty of Arts, Kuwait University http://www.islam-set.com/hip/Abu_Reidah/main.html Accesssed March 17, 2003.

Australian Bureau of Statistics 2002 Causes of death, Australia – 2001. http://www.abs.gov.au/Ausstats/abs@nsf/look upMF/2093DA6935DB138FCA2568A90013 93C9 Accessed March 9, 2003.

Blaxter M 1990 Health & lifestyles. Tavistock/Routledge, London.

Central Intelligence Agency (CIA) 2001 The World Factbook 2001. CIA, Washington DC; Bartleby.com, New York http://www.bartle-by.com/151 Accessed March 7, 2003.

Central Statistical Office 2000 Guide to official statistics. HMSO, London. http://www.statis-tics.gov.uk/statbase/Product.asp?vlnk=1551& More=N Accessed March 17, 2003.

Community Health Endowment of Lincoln 1998 Creating the Healthiest Community in the Nation: Recommendations from the Mayor's Task Force on Lincoln General Sale Proceeds. Community Health Endowment, Lincoln, Nebraska http://www.chelincoln.org/ab_defin.htm Accessed March 17, 2003.

Department of Health and Social Security 1976 Everybody's business. HMSO, London.

Department of Health and Social Security 1980 Inequalities in health: report of a research working group (The Black Report). HMSO, London.

Galli N 1978 Foundations and principles of health education. John Wiley, London

Gideon TryAgain 2003 Capability Oriented Definition of Health. www.tryagain.com/humanbody/capahlth.htm Accessed March 17, 2003.

Goldberg D Williams P 1988 A User's Guide to the General Health Questionnaire. NFER-Nelson, Windsor.

Green AE 1994 The geography of poverty and wealth. Institute for Employment Research, University of Warwick, Warwick.

Health Canada/Santé Canada 2000 Leading causes of death and hospitalisation in Canada (1997). Health Canada/Santé Canada Population and Public Health Branch. http://www.hc-sc.gc.ca/pphb-dgspsp/publi-cat/lcd-pc97/mrt_mf_e.html Accessed March 9, 2003.

Information and Statistics Division (ISD) Scotland 2001 ISD Online – Top 5 Most Common Reasons for Consulting a GP by sex and age group: year ending December 2000. http://www.show.scot.nhs.uk/isd/primary_car e/gmp/pcare_gmp_dia_20008.htm Accessed March 9, 2003.

Khayat MH 1997 Spirituality in the Definition of Health: The World Health Organization's Point of View. http://www.medizin-ethik.ch/publik/spirituality_definition_health. htm Accessed March 17, 2003.

Kirsten W 2001 Health Promotion – An International Phenomenon. National Center for Health Fitness, American University, Washington DC http://216.239.51.100/search?q=cache:lTmK Wt3i4v0C:www.american.edu/academic.dept s/cas/health/iihp/archives/pubsiihpchinawolf.h tml+Greek+definition+health&hl=en&ie=UT F-8 Accessed March 18, 2003.

Levin LS 1977 Health education: moving to centre stage. Connecticut Medicine 39(10): 631-634.

McCormick A, Fleming D, Charlton J 1995 Morbidity Statistics in General Practice, 4th National Study 1991-1992. HMSO, London.

McDowell I Newell C 1996 Measuring Health. A Guide to Rating Scales and Questionnaires Second Edition. Oxford University Press, Oxford.

Mercer P 2000 Justice and Health in the Bible. Lukes Journal 2000 5(4):4-7.

Mitchell R, Shaw M & Dorling D 2000 Inequalities in Life and Death: What if Britain were more equal? The Policy Press, University of Bristol.

NHS Scotland 1999 National Health Service in Scotland: Annual Report 1998-99. Scottish Executive, Edinburgh.

Noble M, Smith G, Avenell D, Smith T, Sharland E 1994 Changing patterns of income and wealth in Oxford and Oldham. Department of Applied Social Studies and Social Research, University of Oxford, Oxford.

Office for National Statistics (ONS) 2002 Mortality Statistics–general–Review of the Registrar General on Deaths in England and Wales, 2000. Series DH1 No. 33. Office for National Statistics, London.

OPCS 1983 Mortality statistics–cause 1982. Series DH2 No 89. HMSO, London.

OPCS 1992 Mortality statistics–serial tables. Review of the Registrar General on deaths in England and Wales, 1841-1990. Series DH1 No 25. HMSO, London.

OPCS 1993 Mortality statistics–cause. Review of the Registrar General on deaths by cause, sex and age, in England and Wales, 1992. HMSO, London.

OPCS 1994 Mortality statistics–general. Review of the Registrar General on deaths in England and Wales, 1992. Series DH1 No 27. HMSO, London.

Population Reference Bureau (PRB) 2000 Women of our World. PRB website: http://www.worldpop.org/prbdata.htm Accessed October 1, 2003.

Population Reference Bureau (PRB) 2003 World Population Data Sheet. PRB website: http://www.worldpop.org/prbdata.htm Accessed October 1, 2003.

Registrar General Scotland 1983 Annual report. HMSO, Edinburgh.

Rose D 1995 Official Social Classifications in the UK.

Social Research Update: Issue nine. Department of Sociology, University of Surrey, Guildford, England http://www.soc.surrey.ac.uk/sru/SRU9.html Accessed March 9, 2003.

Savary LM, O'Connor TJ, Cullen RM, Plummer DM 1970 Listen to love. Regina Press, New York.

Scottish Office Department of Health (SODH) 1998 Working Together for a Healthier Scotland: A Consultation Document, CM 3854. The Stationary Office, Edinburgh.

Scottish Home and Health Department (SHHD) 1991 Health education in Scotland: a national policy statement. St Andrew's House, Edinburgh.

Smith A, Jacobson B (eds) 1988 The nation's health. A strategy for the 1990s. King's Fund, London.

Statistics Division, Department of Health 2002 Mortality Statistics–Cause. Government Statistical Service, London http://www.doh.gov.uk/HPSSS/ Accessed March 22, 2003.

Statistics South Africa 2002 Causes of death in South Africa 1997-2001. Statistics South Africa, Pretoria. http://www.statssa.gov.za Accessed March 9, 2003.

Travis JW (2000) Concepts in Wellness. Wellness Associates, Mill Valley California. http://www.thewellspring.com/Pubs/lw_cont.html Accessed March 20, 2003.

US Department of Health and Human Services 2000 Healthy People 2010. US Department of Health and Human Services, Office of Disease Prevention and Health Promotion, Washington, DC.

Whitehead M 1987 The health divide: inequalities in health in the 1980s. Health Education Council, London.

World Health Organization (WHO) 1947 Constitution. WHO, New York.

WHO 1984 Health promotion. A discussion document on the concept and principles. WHO, Copenhagen.

WHO 2003 WHO Statistics – Mortality Database. WHO, Copenhagen http://www3.who.int/whosis/mort/ Accessed March 28, 2003.

2 Health education concepts and practice

HEALTH EDUCATION APPROACHES AND MODELS

To begin this chapter, it is important to address particular issue about terms, namely the distinction between 'health *education*' and 'health *promotion*', and to clarify how the terms are used in this book. Many people involved in these areas of work see a clear difference between the two terms, usually viewing health promotion as an umbrella term which includes health education plus other approaches to promoting health (e.g. Mackintosh 1996; Norton 1998; Whitehead 2001). Some authors, such as Brown and Piper (1995), take a restricted view of health education, seeing it as persuasion aimed at achieving a specific type of health-related behaviour. Others see health education in a wider view, such as Philips (1995) who takes it as including community empowerment activities. Thus the boundary between health education and health promotion often seems to be blurred, because even writers who make a distinction between the two terms do not seem to agree as to what each term means specifically. Because this book is about *Teaching for Health*, the term 'health education' seems to relate most appropriately to its aim. However, the term is not used here in a narrow sense, but in a sense that encompasses a range of purposes, methods and outcomes of the nurse's teaching. Thus, as will become evident, health education is here taken to include all sorts of teaching contexts and events, from the teaching of the individual patient at the bedside about what his diabetes means or how to take his insulin, to the teaching of families about how to manage a newly disabled family member, to the running of group sessions in a clinic on smoking cessation, to activities aimed at empowering community groups to participate effectively in campaigns about health-related environmental issues. Education is a key element in all of these, and it is accepted that all also have the potential to promote health.

Health education is based upon the assumption that the health status of individuals or communities may be influenced purposefully. Opinions differ about how such influence can and should be achieved, and so the nature of health education varies with the underlying health aspirations of the society in which the health education takes place, the knowledge base and resources available to health educators and the assumptions which are made about the purpose of health education.

Health educators have been described as falling into two groups: those who assume that they have a duty to use persuasive strategies to help people learn new patterns of behaviour, and those who assume that health education is aimed at assisting rather than persuading people to change (Simonds 1977; Tones 1977). It may be that these two positions have reflected differences in the beliefs of the teaching and medical professions (Vuori 1980). More recently, the problem has been addressed by Jones and Naidoo (2000) who refer to work by Beattie (1991) and Foucault (1973) in their discussion. They characterize the 'conservative' model of health persuasion as attempting to promote health by attempting to repair deficits. They contrast this with a community development approach, which they describe as being based on 'assumptions about power and equity and the mobilisation of communities to effect change'. They further point out differences between a 'traditional, medical approach which focuses on the individual and on the treatment of disease' and more radical approaches that are 'linked to Health for All strategies' (Jones & Naidoo 2000, p. 91). Such polarized distinctions help to identify an important ethical issue relating to health education, but they clearly fail to deal with the complexity of the persuasion problem. Health educators remain divided not only on the issue of whether or not to persuade, but also on how persuasion is to be achieved, who needs to be persuaded and how persuasion should be applied.

Health education is a multifaceted activity, employing a variety of means and strategies to deal with the promotion of health in society. Historically its purposes and methods have changed as the health status and needs of society have changed. Rawson and Grigg (1988) described 17 different taxonomies of British health education models. Thus there is a wide range of ways in which models of health education can be categorized and discussed. In this chapter, approaches to health education will be described as:

- the information-giving or medical model
- the educational model
- the propaganda or media model
- the enabling or community development model
- the political model.

These models of health education are summarized in Table 2.1. It should be noted that the models are not entirely discrete; some share certain elements with others, and they do not have to be operated in isolation from each other. The reader should also remember that there are other ways of classifying such theoretical models; the scheme selected here is simply one rational way of organizing such a discussion. As will also be evident, there is a historical dimension to the order of the models.

TABLE 2.1	Models of health education			
Model	**Assumptions**	**Strategy**	**Tactics**	**Role of practitioner**
Medical	The facts will persuade. The advice of experts is highly valued.	Generate and promote clear and simple messages.	Identify cost-effective methods of presenting information. Package the material attractively.	As expert informant, give talks, prepare booklets, exploit new media techniques to improve presentation.
Educational	Education will elicit potential and achieve autonomy. Exploration of values and feelings will activate health action.	Assess learning needs and readiness with reference to the group concerned and relevant research, then generate a systematic planned approach.	Set clear objectives. Identify evaluation criteria. Ensure feedback.	As educator/enabler, lead the person to learning discoveries, set up opportunities to discuss feelings and challenge 'facts'.
Media	People have to be manipulated to value health and adopt a healthy lifestyle. Health can be 'sold'.	Create and provide positive health images. Increase awareness of the impact of disease.	Use role modelling, repetition, rhetoric and fear arousal.	As persuader, present an image and package the message persuasively.
Community development	People have strengths. They will want to use them to improve their health on their terms.	Offer a 'let's get together and talk about this' approach to determine felt needs.	Organize discussion and communication among a wide range of individuals on given health issues to arrive at consensus.	As enabler, help people express discontents, encourage organization to facilitate change, nourish interpersonal relationships.
Political	Change in the institutions and structures of society is needed to improve health. Power, local and national, must be mobilized.	Create an awareness of health issues. Influence the decision-makers.	Lobby politicians. Embarrass anti-health profiteers. Mobilize local support.	As provocateur, provide evidence, draft letters, facilitate action.

The information-giving (medical) model

The information-giving approach is, just as it sounds, an approach that entails providing information for people about health-related matters. It makes use of material and methods such as leaflets, posters, television documentaries, lectures and talks. The stress is upon presenting factual information in a way that makes it interesting and easily understood. Health educators who use information-giving strategies assume that it is their job to present people with facts about health and let them decide for themselves what to think and do about it. The single-minded use of this approach assumes, first of all, that all recipients will understand information presented in a single format. Perhaps more profoundly, it assumes that people make conscious choices about health behaviour and that factual information alone will influence those choices, in other words, that people behave rationally in relation to their health. Clearly, such an assumption may be challenged. It is true that some people make rational choices about health some of the time. However, the cigarette-smoking nurse or doctor and the nibbling weight-watcher provide just two reminders that rationality is not the only influence on health behaviour.

Another problem with the information-giving approach is that what appears rational to one person may appear irrational to another. For instance, it is rational to take time and trouble to care for one's teeth if one wants to keep them for a lifetime. It is equally rational not to spend time, energy and money on dental care if one believes that it is normal to have all one's teeth extracted and replaced with dentures in early middle age, a traditional practice in some cultures. A serious limitation of the information-giving approach to health education is that, on its own, it ignores the question of motivating people to adopt particular health-related behaviour. It assumes that everyone agrees about the meaning and purpose of being healthy and is anxious to achieve 'health'. Further, it ignores the existence of other factors which affect people's beliefs and values and which thus influence their health-related behaviour.

Health professionals can fall into the trap of assuming either that their health values are generally held, or that at the very least, lay people will acknowledge them as the right values since they are based on professional knowledge and expertise. This undue emphasis on rationality, coupled with the assumption that expert authority will be acknowledged (and is necessarily the only correct view), has at times led to heavy reliance by nurses and doctors on the information-giving approach to health education. For this reason, the term 'medical model' has been used to describe this approach (Vuori 1980; Thompson 1983; Ewles & Simnett 1999).

The origins of the medical model of health education in Britain lie in the 19th century, when the main health preoccupation was the control of infectious disease. A parallel concern was the interest of the great reformers in the welfare and social conditions of the working poor. The latter half of the century, a time of great social reform, saw a rapid increase in the use of legislative power to improve living conditions generally and the lot of the poor in particular (Wohl 1983; Smout 1986).

Many of the reformers were men of religion who saw aspiring to good health as the godly thing to do. Self-denial was a prominent theme, as is illustrated by the preface to a little book recording some health lectures given to the people of Edinburgh during the winter of 1880-1881 (Anon 1881) which states:

> The oldest record of man's history tells of a fall in condition from pure greediness of desire. God knows what was lost in early days, but the last, divinest teacher of the world struck again the keynote sounded by divine wisdom at Creation and declared that through self-denial alone we should reach not simply health but Immortal Life.

Such a social context set the scene for health educators to assume responsibility for telling people what to do and what not to do, since they operated in a society in which control of the many by a privileged few was usual. The time was also set for the emergence of doctors as the experts who could tell people about health.

Sanitary and other reforms of the 19th century brought gradual improvements in standards of living, including nutrition. Infectious diseases were combated and disease patterns changed (Smout 1986). During this time, medical and scientific discoveries accelerated and this led to an emphasis on the contribution to health which might be expected from medical science. It seems to have been widely assumed that these new experts should process information for people and make judgements about health on their behalf.

As late as the 1960s in Britain, a report of the Central and Scottish Health Services Councils, known widely as the Cohen Report (Ministry of Health 1964), reflected medical domination over health matters. This view is evident in the statement that the four main contributions to health of health education were:

(i)   Advice about specific preventive measures

(ii) Education with a view to inculcating habits and attitudes which will promote health and prevent disease

(iii) Education to understand the need for community health measures and support them

(iv) Education to seek advice from the doctor at an early stage for certain conditions. (p. 13)

The tone of this extract implies that what is meant by 'education' in this context is 'instruction' or 'direction'.

The impact of the medical model was that health education developed as a tool of preventive medicine, concentrating on the prevention of disease rather than emphasizing the more positive aspects of health. Health education messages based solely on the medical concept of being at risk of disease are often negative, threatening and authoritarian in tone. More recent thinking among health educators is that such messages achieve only limited results. A further danger of single-minded operation of the medical model can be the adoption of an attitude that the professional or medical view is the only credible view. This attitude may lead the health professional to ignore or discount other legitimate views. It can also lead to confusion in the minds of members of the public when the information being disseminated by some 'experts' differs from information being disseminated by others, as has happened recently in the UK with messages about the safety of the 'single-jab' measles-mumps-rubella immunization or the safety of genetically modified (GM) foods.

ACTIVITY 2.1

Can you think of examples, in your own life, of times when you were told what to do for your health, by a health professional? This might have been your GP, a school nurse, a health visitor or the like. What was the content of the advice or instruction? How did you respond to this health education? Did it influence your behaviour, beliefs or attitudes?

The educational model

The educational approach to health education challenges the naive assumptions of the medical model by acknowledging that beliefs, values and feelings may influence what people are prepared to do about health. This approach promotes the idea that the health educator should take the meaning of the term 'education' to heart, considering it as a means of leading toward discovery rather than instilling facts. It became known as the educational model because it adopts the rhetoric and methodology of educationalists (Vuori 1980; Thompson 1983). The educational approach emphasizes that health education should be concerned with affective (emotional) as well as cognitive (intellectual) aspects of learning. It introduces the idea that each individual has a 'health learning career' (Tones 1979) from the cradle to the grave, and proposes that health education activity should capitalize on the particular opportunities which arise for motivating the individual. Instances might include the chance to shape attitudes of the child while at primary school or to change attitudes of the adult during life crises such as hospitalization.

With this approach, much of the activity is directed at helping the person develop skills in decision-making and in clarifying values and beliefs about health. A full range of educational methods may be employed, but often there is emphasis on group work.

Nonetheless, this model, too, has its limitations. The educational approach rests on more than mere provision of information. It may provide an acceptable and successful way to change individuals, and it encompasses a dimension beyond that of the medical model alone. It does not, however, change the structures in society which perpetuate ill health. Although it is suitable for many nursing situations, particularly some types of patient education, if applied alone it may be too limited to bring about meaningful change in health status differentials. Consider, for example, the social class inequalities in health that were mentioned in Chapter 1. However successful the health educator is in enhancing people's understandings about health and health behaviour, education alone cannot change their social class, or the life context which that social class implies.

Another limitation of the educational model is that it may bring individuals into conflict with existing value systems. For instance, following school programmes in health education, children may question their family's dietary habits or their parents' smoking. The approach needs a parallel support system and in practice this can be difficult to provide.

The educational model of health education evolved from the 1950s onwards out of a growing recognition that health has social as well as medical aspects. When the World Health Organization (WHO) was constituted in 1947, it published its now well-known definition referring to health as 'not merely the absence of disease' (WHO 1947). A few years later, the first report of an expert committee on health education of the public (WHO 1954) acknowledged that:

> The first problem of concern to the community may not be directly related to health. It may be one of agriculture, transportation, irrigation, housing or accident prevention, or of mere subsistence. Cooperation for health begins with the problem of immediate interest, assists in its solu-

tion and then is ready to help on health problems as they become of serious concern to the community. (p. 5)

This view that lay and professional priorities in relation to health might differ was coupled with the acknowledgement that health messages might be rejected unless they took account of the existing beliefs, attitudes and feelings of the people to whom they were directed. The report laid great stress on how people learn, and presented health education as an activity planned to take account of the complexity of human learning:

> Health education, like general education, is concerned with change in the knowledge, feelings and behaviour of people. In its most usual form it concentrates on developing such health practices as are believed to bring about the best possible state of well-being. In order to be effective, its planning methods and procedures must take into consideration both the processes by which people acquire knowledge, change their feelings and modify their behaviour and the factors that influence such changes. (p. 8)

In addition, it was emphasized that health education should be less concerned with 'information-giving' and 'publicity' and should make more use of educational techniques and theories. Two types of educational method were distinguished: didactic methods, which assume that the learner is an empty vessel into which information is poured; and Socratic methods, which assume that people already possess information, feelings, interests and beliefs which will affect the learning process and which therefore have to be taken into account in planning health education.

Emphasis was laid upon Socratic or 'two-way' methods, and there was concern to ensure participation of people in the learning process, the rationale being that active learning is generally more effective than passive learning. There was also an assumption that involvement in the learning process would motivate the learner.

The nature of the educational model of health education which was promoted during the 1960s and 1970s is clearly reflected in statements made by Pisharoti (1975) about his understanding of the term health education. He described it as having '*knowledge, attitude* and *behaviour components*' and being aimed at '*individual, family* and *community behaviour* and their *interaction* patterns'. He also stressed that health education was a '*process*' rather than a single procedure, and that '*learning* takes place through the *efforts of learners*', while the health educator '*provides* the circumstances in which the learning takes place' (p. 5).

ACTIVITY 2.2

Are you aware of having received health education at school? If so, in what subjects or classes did it take place? What topics were covered? What methods of teaching were used (e.g. lectures, group discussions, projects, diaries)? How did you respond to this health education? Did it influence your behaviour, beliefs or attitudes?

The propaganda (media) model

The educational model's assumption that the opportunity to explore information, values and feelings results in changed health-related behaviour is borne out for some, but by no means all, of the population. The question of how to motivate change in health behaviour has became an increasing concern throughout the 1960s and 1970s, despite increasing sophistication of health education planning and methodology, and it remains a concern to the present day. The educational model stresses the importance of developing the individual's skills in relation to recognizing health options and making informed choices, but the tension between the desire to allow the individual the responsibility for his own decisions and the need to persuade him to act wisely, is reflected in this quotation from a WHO (1969) report on the planning and evaluation of health education:

> The focus of health education is on people and on action. In general, its aims are to persuade people to adopt and sustain healthful life practices, to use judiciously and wisely the health services available to them, and to take their own decisions, both individually and collectively, to improve their health status and environment. (p. 8)

The need to confront the problem of motivation has meant that there are always some people who argue that a propaganda approach to health education is necessary. This approach involves the use of means such as poster campaigns and mass media for the purpose of persuasion. It assumes that the health educator knows best about health and has a duty to persuade others to

| FIGURE 2.1 | *Health education media campaign slogans* |

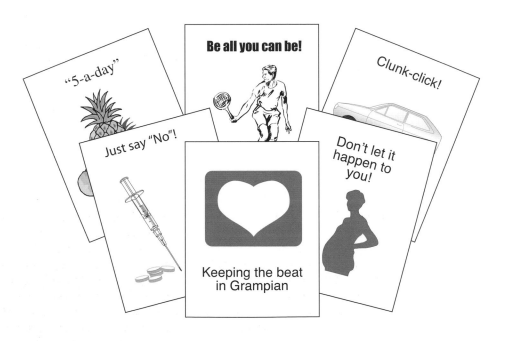

adopt values and practices which are known to be beneficial in combating disease. (Note here the element of similarity with the assumptions of the medical model.)

Health educators who utilize propaganda argue that it is naive to assume the free choice of individuals in a society bombarded with anti-health messages. They claim that the individual should be persuaded to adopt good health practices for his own good and for the good of others. Propagandists typically concentrate on emotional aspects of the argument and are less concerned about logic and the facts of the case. Because modern propagandizing has made much use of television in particular, this approach may be referred to as a media model of health education. The media model assumes that there exists a mass and homogeneous audience of people and that 'health' may be marketed in much the same way as other products. Clearly, both these assumptions may be challenged.

Apart from the ethical issues it raises, propagandizing is criticized by some health educators on the grounds that its effects are short-lived. Motivation springing from emotional response may not be maintained once the stimulus is removed. The impressive but short-lived successes of fear-based appeals in some 'stop smoking' television programmes provide an example.

Another limitation of the media model is that often, of necessity, it promotes simplistic messages about very complex health issues. Catchy slogans (see Figure 2.1) may be remembered, so to that extent they can be useful, but by themselves they are seldom able to convey real information. It may also be claimed that via the media model, health education may be powerfully, and even dishonestly, directed exclusively at the individual, placing an unreasonable share of the responsibility for health upon him or her without providing any support or reference system and thus contributing to what has been described as 'blaming the victim' (WHO 1981).

In more recent applications, the media model of health education has incorporated attempts by health educators to influence the presentation of health issues in media outlets such as women's magazines and television 'soap operas', in addition to the traditional approach of advertising health images or messages. In recent British soap operas, for example, story lines have included issues such as HIV/AIDS, breast cancer and mental illness. Often after a particularly emotional episode involving such a topic, a message is broadcast giving viewers telephone help-line numbers, addresses or websites they can use if they 'have been affected' by the material they have seen in the episode.

ACTIVITY 2.3

While you watch television over two or three evenings, look for examples of health and anti-health messages. Health messages might be in the form of health education 'adverts', for example, or in issues that appear in the story lines of dramas or soap operas, such as those described in the text. Anti-health messages might be in commercial advertisements, but they can also be found in virtually any type of programme. Sometimes they are blatant, but sometimes they are very subtle, so keep your eyes and ears open! Jot down a note of any such messages you find. Do you think you are influenced by them? If so, how, and how much, do they influence your behaviour, beliefs or attitudes? Are you aware of any other types of media sources by which health and/or anti-health messages are delivered?

The enabling (community development) model

The medical, educational and media approaches to health education all, to a greater or lesser degree, assume that the responsibility for health education and the skills and resources needed for the process rest with professionals. Enabling strategies are based on a different assumption: that people have strengths and abilities which they will be willing to contribute, on their own terms, to the process of learning about and achieving health.

Educators often label themselves 'enablers'. It is part of the rhetoric of educationalists to describe themselves as working 'with' rather than 'on' people. So 'enabling' is an old idea in health education. It does, however, have some new connotations.

Since Illich (1971, 1974) questioned the wisdom of institutionalizing both health and education, there has been growing concern about the 'medicalization of life' – in other words, about the extent to which health care experts generally, and doctors in particular, have influenced the interpretation of the term 'health' (Wilson 1975; McKeown 1976; Kennedy 1981).

The main thrust of these challenges is that health systems can no longer devote themselves exclusively to providing medical and related care while ignoring all other influences upon health. The complex and costly health care systems of the Western world have been challenged as socially irrelevant and there is growing realization that the optimizing of health will depend on achieving lay-professional partnerships in care and on coordinating the activities of health workers with workers in the social and economic sectors.

An international conference held in Alma Ata, USSR, in September 1978 (WHO 1978) declared it obvious that the 'health sector' would not achieve health by working alone. It urged all governments to bring health care systems as close as possible to where people live and work, emphasizing full and organized community participation. The conference proposed that traditionally separate levels of primary, secondary and tertiary care should be joined in a new approach in which the caring tasks and roles would be closely geared to needs as defined by the people themselves. From this conference came the broad but ambitious statement of a goal: 'Health for all by the year 2000' – a phrase which has become well known during the years since the Alma Ata conference.

For health education, the particular challenge has been to move from thinking primarily about the prevention of disease, a medical bias, to the promotion of health based on people's needs. In a paper outlining how health for all could be achieved in Europe (WHO 1981), the change was described thus:

> Health education has, in theory, gone far beyond an approach that seeks to improve health by changing individual behaviour without taking into account the environment which enables or reinforces the possibilities of such behaviour change. Health education has come a long way from just 'blaming the victim' to a concept of developing awareness of health and providing the opportunities for more informed choices. One of its main concepts is now that of the individual in health care as a competent actor in a community setting. (p. 1)

Recent initiatives in enabling strategies have sprung from a concern to deal with the economic and political realities of health and to address accusations

TABLE 2.2	Trends in the development of health education concepts and practice		
Underlying health aspirations	Prevailing purposes	Scientific bases emphasized	Methods in use
1850–1950 (approximately)			
Reduce infectious diseases, improve standards of hygiene, improve nutrition	Inform about health hazards, propagandize about the benefits of prevention	Medical science	Leaflets, posters, talks, blackboard, films
1950s–1970s			
Prevent and cope with chronic disease	Acknowledge social aspects of health, help people take informed decisions about health options	Behavioural science	As above, plus more sophisticated audiovisual aids, group work, decision-making/ problem-solving exercises, advertising, use of TV
Late 1970s onwards			
Shifting emphasis from medical domination to lay participation in care and decision-making	Enable participation in health care, acknowledge alternative forms of health care	Firmer adherence to both scientific bases, with emphasis on making technical acknowledge accessible and increasing concern about evaluation	As above, plus growing interest in non-directive techniques, and ever more sophisticated technology such as the Internet

that traditional health education approaches have only been effective with the middle classes. One such new approach to health education comes from the theoretical background of community development.

The community development idea holds out the hope that it will be possible to reduce factors which alienate large numbers of people in a modern industrialized society and achieve a greater sense of community involvement. There are many ways of defining what is meant by community, but one approach is to accept that communities will be geographically determined and that everyone within a given locality will be considered as belonging to the 'community', so that no state of 'them and us' can exist. Barriers, whether lay-professional or any other, thus disappear. The professional worker views all parts of the community as part of the client system and accepts that only goals which are mutually agreed may be pursued. Clients or patients are viewed as citizens who possess strengths and who are capable of participating in a problem-solving approach to achieving health.

The community development approach is one of the younger approaches in health education, but evidence exists which suggests that it is having an impact on the general tenor of health education. The trends in this development can be seen in Table 2.2. On a superficial level, a difference can be seen in the terminology which has gained favour in recent years. The tendency to use the term 'health promotion' in place of 'health education' itself implies a change in

| TABLE 2.3 | | *Contrasting approaches to health education practice* | | |

		Directive ←——————————————→ Non-directive		
		Educator (at times with the help of the learner(s))	*Group members*	*Enabler (often by asking questions)*
	Step 1	Identify and describe the target group	Some dissatisfaction or need for change felt but not expressed	Stimulate people to think what their health concerns/ needs are
	Step 2	Assess needs	Begin to be aware of needs	Stimulate thought about changes that would reduce concerns, meet needs
	Step 3	Set objectives	Recognize specific changes needed	Stimulate people to consider what they could do to achieve changes
	Step 4	Plan a teaching programme	In specific terms decide for or against trying to achieve changes or meet needs	If necessary help people decide how to organize for the tasks they have decided to undertake
	Step 5	Choose teaching methods and materials	Plan what to do and how to do it	Stimulate people as necessary to allocate tasks and decide on a timetable
	Step 6	Carry out the teaching programme	Carry out the plan	Stimulate people to consider potential problems and plan avoiding action
	Step 7	Evaluate	Assess what they have achieved and express their reactions	

emphasis. In addition, terms such as 'empowerment' and 'self-help' indicate a shift away from the professional focus that existed so strongly in the past, towards a focus on individuals from their own perspective.

An important difference in the conduct of health education and health promotion activities is the extent to which non-directive techniques are used. Community development takes a different starting point from community provision, in which the health education service is provided on the basis of professional identification of needs. The community development model thus challenges traditional approaches and complex professionally-devised health education planning models. Adherents of the approach claim that it offers the opportunity to improve human relationships, develop problem-solving skills and increase self-esteem in a way that will make health education relevant to multiply-deprived groups in society who are widely believed to have been failed by the traditional medical and educational models. The tactical and planning approaches of the educational model and the community development model are contrasted in Table 2.3.

The political action model

The idea that there is a need for political action to achieve societal improvements that will impinge on the health status of individuals is not new. However, the role of health education in generating political action for health has taken on new dimensions in recent years. The purpose of this approach is to stimulate communities to seek their rights, including their rights to health. The underlying assumption of the political action approach is that underprivileged communities cannot be expected to operate on their own behalf and require assistance to engage in conflict with powerful authorities.

Given the inequalities in health that continue to exist in Britain (DHSS 1980; Whitehead 1987; Blaxter 1990; Clark et al 2004), it is increasingly likely that health educators will be challenged to be involved in political activity to help people achieve health. At the very least, some people will feel that health educators should play a part in bringing inconsistencies and inequalities in health care provision to the forefront of the political agenda for discussion. Others take the view that health educators should act as patient or client advocates, given the present unequal distribution of power in relation to health.

The exercise of political power to achieve health is a tradition stemming from the 19th century when many improvements in health were achieved by the exercise of legislative power. Today, fiscal and legal controls, such as taxation on alcohol and tobacco, penalties for not using seat belts, legislation for health and safety at work, and regulations aimed at reducing vehicle emissions are used as mechanisms to reduce the toll of modern problems of ill health. Additionally, there is increasing emphasis on the power of people in local communities (Kickbush 1983; Smithies & Webster 1998) and on the political role of the health educator in releasing such local potential.

In 1986, an international conference resulted in the Ottawa Charter for Health Promotion (WHO 1986). Within the Charter it was stressed that governments at all levels have responsibility for the health consequences of their policy decisions. The philosophy implied by this is, in a sense, in opposition to the 'victim-blaming' that may be inherent in some interpretations of the other models. That is, instead of concentrating only on the individual's need to adopt attitudes and behaviours that will foster good health, the political action model acknowledges the influence of the social and physical environment on health in ways that are beyond the control of individuals. Furthermore, it demonstrates the need for health to be a matter of concern for a wide range of

ACTIVITY 2.4

Are you aware of any community development activities going on in your community? If so, what health issues are involved, and what sort of activity is taking place? If not, can you identify health education/promotion issues (in the broadest sense of 'health') that might usefully be addressed using a community development model? How might the issues be approached?

ACTIVITY 2.5

Identify two or three health problems that might be solved by political action rather than by modification of individuals' lifestyles. For each of these issues, consider the following questions: What type of action would be needed to bring about necessary improvement? What levels or agencies of government would need to be involved? What arguments might be made on both sides of the issue? How might a campaign seek to apply effective pressure on government to achieve the necessary change?

government agencies. It is not only the traditional health sector whose policies either contribute to or detract from the protection and improvement of public health. Almost any government agency's activities have an impact on some aspect of health.

Reflection on the models

A summary comparison of the five models just described can be seen in Table 2.1. The astute reader will have noted that not all health education is account-ed for in this scheme of models. Although some of the models deliberately avoid placing the health or education professional in a controlling position, all of them assume the presence of *some* professional in *some* guise, if only in an enabling capacity. This leaves out, for example, the sort of health education that goes on, and has gone on for hundreds of years, within families and com-munities – the parent teaching a child to wash hands after using the toilet, the mother explaining menstruation to her daughter, the father having a chat about 'the birds and the bees' with his son, the adult taking on the coaching of a young people's sports team in the neighbourhood, and so on. Obviously, such everyday health education/promotion activities are important and should not be discounted. Nor should they be ignored as being irrelevant to the health educator's work; there are ways in which formal health education has an influ-ence on such efforts, though often indirectly, and there are ways in which such efforts have implications for formal health education.

It was mentioned earlier that the models discussed in this chapter need not necessarily be seen or operated in isolation from one another. Health educa-tors often use strategies that draw on more than one model. It is easy to see, for example, how the community development model and the political action model might be combined within one campaign. A community may identify its own health needs, and the health educator might take an enabling role in this, and might then support community action to try to achieve appropriate changes in political policy.

HEALTH EDUCATION/PROMOTION SERVICES IN THE UK

Ever since man first recognized that aspect of life we call health, there have been health teachers, some amateur, some with more clearly defined status as experts or professionals. Depending on country and culture, the expert health teacher may be a wise man, witch doctor, religious leader, health care professional, school teacher or union official. In Britain today, a variety of people consider themselves to be professional health educators. A health education/health promotion service is provided for the sick as well as for the healthy, and health teaching is carried out by a range of agents in a variety of places, but the present discussion focuses on the health education and promotion services that have evolved within the National Health Service.

National organizations

The history of health education is as old as mankind, but it is only necessary to look as far back as the beginning of the last century to trace the development of our modern health education service. At the end of the 19th century, and for the first half of the 20th, there was widespread belief that medical science would in time cure all ills and ensure the health of the population. Early health education services developed out of a desire to promote that belief and to encourage people in the use of new services such as antenatal clinics. Local staff, often health visitors or public health doctors, prepared posters and exhibitions and gave public lectures to advertise the services.

By the 1920s it was realized that such ad hoc local arrangements were costly and that duplicated efforts were wasteful. In the UK, Sir Allen Daley, then the Medical Officer of Health for Bootle, in Lancashire, began to press for the formation of a central body to be responsible for the development of health education materials. He argued that a central body with good funding could coordinate efforts and do a great deal to promote the development of health education. In 1924, he presented a paper entitled *The Organisation of Propaganda in the Interests of Public Health* to the annual meeting of the Society of Medical Officers of Health (Daley 1959).

This paper aroused great interest in the idea of a central body and in health education generally, but some local authorities were worried that when accounts were audited, questions would be asked about spending money on health education. There were those who questioned whether or not it was legal to spend public money to persuade the public to adopt particular types of behaviour. A deputation went to Neville Chamberlain, who was Minister of Health in Baldwin's government (Thomson 1965), to persuade him that there was need for legal support for health education. This subsequently was granted in Section 67 of the 1925 Public Health Act. Health education was now sanctioned in law and the movement towards a central organization could proceed.

By 1927, the Central Council for Health Education had been constituted, with responsibility for developing health education in England and Wales. Twenty years later, a parallel Scottish organization was formed, the Scottish Council for Health Education. These Councils organized lecture tours, study days, exhibitions and health fairs. They also produced a wide range of audiovisual materials for use in health education and provided a backup service for anyone, amateur or professional, concerned with developing health education services on a local basis.

The 1950s brought a series of reports on health education produced by the WHO (1954, 1958). These reflected growing international awareness of new challenges to health education, in particular the need to respond to the realization that modern diseases arose from the very fabric of society and were inextricably linked with the lifestyle of individuals. There was growing appreciation that health education might be used as an instrument of planned social change, rather than merely as the information arm of preventive medicine.

One British response to these new challenges was to set up, in the 1960s, a Joint Committee of the Central and Scottish Health Services, with a remit to investigate health education needs and provision in the United Kingdom. The resulting Cohen Report (Ministry of Health 1964) laid the basis for national and local health education services. The Report recommended that there should be established, in England and Wales, a strong central body which would promote the development of health education, identify priorities and secure support from all possible sources, commercial and voluntary as well as medical, and assist local authorities and other agencies in the conduct of local programmes. Such a body would also be required to foster the training of specialist health educators, to promote the training in health education of doctors, nurses, teachers and dentists, and to evaluate the results of health education. A parallel body for Scotland was also recommended, which would absorb the health education functions of the Scottish Home and Health Department and the Scottish Council for Health Education.

Following the Cohen Report, two new central agencies for health education were formed in 1968. The Health Education Council took over the responsibilities for England and Wales previously exercised by the Central Council. In Scotland, the new organization, the Scottish Health Education Unit, operated in parallel with the Scottish Council for Health Education until they were both disbanded in 1980 with the formation of the Scottish Health Education Group.

The Health Education Council (HEC) and the Scottish Health Education Group (SHEG) had very similar remits. In general, their activities included helping to determine health education priorities, mounting national campaigns, sponsoring research and surveys, and producing health information and audiovisual materials. Both organizations acted as centres of expertise, providing a source of epidemiological, sociological and psychological data for a wide variety of people involved in health education. They promoted health education training for health care professionals, cooperated with local health and education authorities and maintained contacts with a wide range of voluntary organizations with a concern for health education.

Within the past two decades, both the HEC and SHEG have been replaced by a succession of new agencies. Separate health education or promotion agencies have been established in England, Scotland, Wales and Northern Ireland.

England

In England, the Health Education Authority (HEA) took over the responsibilities of the Health Education Council on 1 April 1987. The HEA was a Special Authority of the National Health Service. Its mission was 'to ensure that by the year 2000 the people of England are more knowledgeable, better motivated and more able to acquire and maintain good health' (HEA July 1994). Its main functions were detailed in Statutory Instrument 1987 No 6 as:

(a) advising the Secretary of State for Health on matters relating to health education activity;

(b) undertaking health education activity;

(c) for that purpose planning and carrying out national and regional or local programmes or other activities in cooperation with health authorities, family practitioner committees, local authorities and local education authorities, voluntary organisations and other persons or bodies concerned with health education;

(d) sponsoring research and evaluation in relation to health education;

(e) assisting the provision of appropriate training in health education;

(f) preparing, publishing or distributing material relevant to health education;

(g) providing a national centre of information and advice on health education.

In addition to these functions which it was to fulfil for England, the HEA was also given responsibility for mass-media education on AIDS throughout the United Kingdom (HEA July 1994).

The members of the Board of the HEA were appointed for terms of up to four years by the Secretary of State for Health. The health education strategy adopted for England by the HEA was based on the assessment of the nation's health needs found in the White Paper *The Health of the Nation: A Strategy for Health in England* (Department of Health 1992), which was presented to Parliament in July 1992. Within the White Paper, five key areas for action were identified, and these can be seen in Box 2.1. National targets were then laid out in relation to each of these key areas. The place of health education within the role of the NHS in achieving the health targets was stated within the White Paper:

> The NHS will improve health education at local level, so that people are able to make informed decisions about their own health and that of their families. The Department of Health and the NHS Management Executive are reviewing with NHS Authorities and the Health Education Authority the role of health authorities in health education, and in particular the way in which authorities are supported by the HEA. The results of this review will be available by the autumn, and a campaign of action to improve health education activity by the NHS will be developed for implementation by 1993. (DoH 1992 p. 36, para. 4.12)

An operational plan was put in place which took account of the stated key areas and targets as well as specifying other areas in which progress would be sought. These included immunization, parent education, and health education for specific groups, namely black and ethnic-minority groups, elderly people and women (HEA 1993).

BOX 2.1	*Key areas for action – England Health of the Nation, DoH 1992*
	■ Coronary heart disease and stroke
	■ Cancers
	■ Mental illness
	■ HIV/AIDS and sexual health
	■ Accidents

In 2000, there was yet another agency change in England, with the HEA closing and being replaced by the Health Development Agency (HDA). The government announced the establishment of the HDA in the White Paper *Saving Lives: Our Healthier Nation* (DoH 1999/2003) that outlined the 1999 public health strategy for England. The HDA's role was based on the aims set out in that White Paper, which were 'to improve the health of everyone, particularly the worst off, taking into account the social, economic and environmental factors affecting health'. 'Health improvement' has become a familiar phrase in discussions about the nation's health. The HDA's particular role in achieving this includes gathering evidence of what works, advising on good practice, and supporting those working to improve the public health (HDA 2003). Comparing its intentions with those of earlier White Papers and strategies, *Saving Lives* set what were described as 'tougher but attainable targets in priority areas' (DoH 1999). These were, by the year 2010:

- *Cancer*: to reduce the death rate in people under 75 by at least a fifth
- *Coronary heart disease and stroke*: to reduce the death rate in people under 75 by at least two fifths
- *Accidents*: to reduce the death rate by at least a fifth and serious injury by at least a tenth
- *Mental illness*: to reduce the death rate from suicide and undetermined injury by at least a fifth. (DoH 1999/2003)

The relevance of these priority targets to the UK mortality statistics described in Chapter 1 is evident.

A number of other important points are emphasised in *Saving Lives*. For example, it stresses the need to tackle smoking, which is described as 'the single biggest preventable cause of poor health' (DoH 1999/2003). It focuses on issues of health inequality, indicating that high standards of health and care should be for everyone, not just for the privileged. It singles out AIDS and variant Creutzfeldt-Jakob disease, two new health problems that do not presently cause large numbers of deaths in the UK but might pose a greater public health problem in future if they are not addressed promptly.

A continuing trend that is evident in *Saving Lives* is the location of a greater amount of responsibility for health within the community. A share of the responsibility for health improvement is devolved to local authorities and primary care groups and trusts. The White Paper announces the setting up of particular 'Healthy Citizens' programmes, including:

- NHS Direct – a nurse-led telephone helpline and Internet service providing information and advice on health
- Health Skills programmes – for people to help themselves and others
- Expert Patients programmes – to help people manage their own illnesses.

Encouraged by such programmes, citizens are to play a greater role in promoting and improving their own health.

In addition to focusing on the key targets mentioned above, the White Paper states that the government will target other important health issues, including sexual health, drugs, alcohol, food safety, water fluoridation and communicable diseases (DoH 1999/2003).

Wales

The Health Promotion Authority for Wales (HPA) took over the Welsh component of the health education/promotion work of the HEC in 1987. The HPA was a Special Health Authority, and its members were appointed by the Secretary of State for Wales (HPA 1990c). Its mission was 'to provide national leadership, support and services for the promotion of health and the prevention of disease for the population of Wales so as to achieve the greatest good for the greatest number' (HPA 1990a p. 16).

The overall strategy for Wales for the 1990s was signalled in a document from the Welsh Office in 1989 (Welsh Health Planning Forum 1989). A reassessment of the existing pattern of health care services was to be guided by three key themes of strategic direction focusing on:

- Health gain
- People centred services
- Effective use of resources (p. 13).

The notion of 'health gain' was to be adopted as the criterion for judging the effectiveness of any activity.

In the following year, in a trio of booklets on *Health for All in Wales*, the HPA published details of the health promotion strategy for the following 5-15 years (HPA 1990a, 1990b, 1990c). The strategy was detailed under four aims within which 26 action areas were specified, as can be seen in Box 2.2.

After devolution transferred certain government functions from the UK level to Scotland and Wales in 1999, health education and promotion in Wales became the responsibility of the Health Promotion Division of the National Assembly for Wales. In 2001, that body published a document entitled *Promoting health and well being: Implementing the national health promotion*

BOX 2.2	*Strategic aims and action areas – Wales* Health for All in Wales, HPA 1990c

Disease prevention	*Health skills*
■ Cardiovascular diseases	■ Knowledge
■ Cancers	■ Attitudes
■ Injuries	■ Self-confidence
■ Maternal and child health	■ Coping and relationships
■ Respiratory diseases	■ Parenting
■ Sexual health	■ Safety and first-aid
■ Mental distress and illness	■ Self-help and mutual support
■ Physical disability and handicap	
■ Dental and oral health	
Healthy lifestyles	*Healthy environments*
■ Smoking	■ Families
■ Alcohol and drugs	■ Communities
■ Nutrition	■ Work and workplace
■ Physical exercise	■ Natural environments
■ Stress and violent behaviour	■ Housing and habitats

strategy (Health Promotion Division 2001). The strategy incorporated five priorities for improving health in Wales:

- Helping communities to develop a shared responsibility for health and to take action to improve people's health
- Promoting healthier lifestyles as part of wider action to address the social and economic factors that affect people's health
- Better communication on health issues – improved quality of information and people's access to it
- Developing the tools, resources and skills for health promotion
- Ensuring action is effective (p. 5).

It will be noted that these priorities are quite general and do not indicate specific health targets. Embedded within the document there is emphasis on the need to tackle smoking, sexual health, healthy eating, physical activity, substance misuse and issues related to older people. Other areas that are mentioned include mental health, oral health, pregnant mothers and babies (especially breastfeeding), the health of people in prisons, and accidents and injuries. Targeted programmes are to be set up which will act as vehicles for the prevention of heart disease and cancers (Health Promotion Division 2001).

Scotland

In 1989, the Scottish Home and Health Department commissioned a firm of management consultants to carry out a fundamental review of health education within Scotland (SHHD 1989). This review led to a number of recommendations, including the following:

- The SHHD should support and continue the move away from concentrating on health education towards focusing on health promotion, within which health education would be one of three components, the other two being prevention and health policy.

BOX 2.3	*Health education target areas – Scotland* Health Education in Scotland, SOHHD 1991

- Coronary heart disease
- Cancers
- Mental illness
- HIV/AIDS
- Accidents
- Dental and oral health
- Smoking
- Alcohol misuse
- Drug misuse (pp. 8–12)

- Responsibility for health promotion should be placed under a single division, and should be removed from the Common Services Agency structure and placed solely with SHEG.
- The SHHD should prepare and disseminate a policy statement on health education/promotion.

Following these recommendations, the Scottish Office Home and Health Department (SOHHD), as it was then called, published a consultation document. This was succeeded by the policy document, *Health Education in Scotland: A National Policy Statement* in March 1991. Health education target areas specified in this document can be seen in Box 2.3. As had been foretold in the consultation document, the Policy Statement also indicated a change in the national agency for health education:

> The Health Education Board for Scotland will be established, from 1 April 1991, as a Special Health Board under Section 28 of the National Health Service and Community Care Act 1990, as the successor to the Scottish Health Education Group. It will be the national centre for health education expertise and information; for the production and supply of materials; for the development of training; and for advice and assistance for local and national organisations. It will undertake health education programmes at a national level, and give a lead to the health education effort in Scotland. The Board's role will necessitate liaison, coordination and close collaboration with other UK, Scottish and local bodies involved in health education. (SOHHD 1991 p. 15)

In 1992, the Scottish Office published a policy statement on health entitled *Scotland's Health: A challenge to us all*. This statement set out a range of initiatives and targets to promote better health. It pointed out that among the developed countries of the world, Scotland had the highest rate of deaths from heart, stroke and circulatory diseases, the highest rate of deaths from cancer, and the poorest life expectancy for both males and females (SOHHD 1992). In support of the policy statement, the Scottish Office also produced a booklet for the public, *Scotland's Health: A challenge to you* (SOHHD undated). Both the policy statement and the booklet emphasized personal behaviour, especially smoking, bad diet, alcohol misuse and lack of exercise. They also focused attention on safe sex, drug misuse (including notions of harm minimization), safety issues in the home, road safety, and prevention of tooth decay (SOHHD 1992 & undated). As can be seen by comparing these with Box 2.3, these health target areas echoed those in the health education policy document.

As of April 2003, the Health Education Board for Scotland (HEBS) is being replaced by NHS Health Scotland. This new special health board will be created through the merger of HEBS and the Public Health Institute of Scotland (PHIS). HEBS and PHIS will continue to operate separately for a period until the merger is fully accomplished.

Northern Ireland

The Health Promotion Agency for Northern Ireland was set up in 1990. It is a special agency of the Department of Health, Social Services and Public Safety.

Its role is to direct and coordinate regional health promotion programmes. It does this by providing publicity, resources, training and research, as well as by supporting local Health and Social Services Boards and voluntary agencies throughout the province. The Agency's mission is 'To make health a top priority for everyone in Northern Ireland' (Health Promotion Agency 2003).

The central importance of health education and promotion was made clear in the Regional Strategy published by the Northern Ireland Department of Health and Personal Social Services for 1992-1997 (DHPSS 1993). Four main themes were identified which set the direction for developments across the services over the period concerned:

- a greater emphasis on health promotion and disease prevention
- the continued improvement of acute hospital services
- a shift from institutional care to care in the community
- targeting health and social need. (p. 12)

Within the document eight key areas of concern were identified to be given priority; these can be seen in Box 2.4. It is interesting to note the relative prominence of children in this list, as compared with the key areas noted for the other countries of the United Kingdom. A reason for this may be the high birth rate in Northern Ireland – one of the highest in Europe (DHPSS 1993 p. 37). Figures from the 2001 census continue to show that children under 16 years of age represent 24% of the Northern Ireland population, as compared with the UK as a whole where the figure is 20% (McKenna 2003).

The areas specified for attention in relation to health promotion in the 1993 Regional Strategy were, as would be expected, related to the identification and reduction of major preventable causes of ill health. They are shown in Box 2.4. A visit to the Agency's website (www.healthpromotionagency.org.uk) in 2003 indicates that the priority areas for attention have altered somewhat. They are listed as nutrition, physical activity, drug and alcohol misuse, smoking, mental health and sexual health. It is interesting that the prominence of children is not apparent in this list. However, at another point the website offers 'areas of work', and the list there includes breastfeeding, children and young people, and parents and children.

BOX 2.4   *Key areas of concern and areas for attention – Northern Ireland* Regional Strategy for *Northern Ireland, DHSS 1993*

Key areas of concern	*Areas for attention*
■ Maternal and child health	■ Cigarette smoking
■ Child care	■ Healthy nutrition
■ Accidents and trauma	■ High blood pressure
■ Physical and sensory disability	■ Physical activity
■ Mental health	■ Alcohol misuse
■ Circulatory diseases	■ HIV and AIDS
■ Cancers	■ Quality of the environment (pp. 15-19)
■ Respiratory diseases (p. 35)	

The 1993 Regional Strategy also addressed the broader role of the Department in relation to health promotion. It acknowledged the need for coordination of action in all matters that relate to health, not just those that fell directly within the scope of the Department of Health and Personal Social Services. It suggested that in this respect, the service agencies within the Department needed to act as advocates of health. It noted the lack of a central mechanism for promoting the health of the public in Northern Ireland and signalled its intention to 'initiate discussions aimed at establishing an inter-Departmental group to consider public health issues and to work together to protect and improve the health of the people in Northern Ireland' (DHPSS 1993 p. 19).

| BOX 2.5 | *Contact details for agencies responsible for health education in the UK* |

For England:

Health Development Agency

Holborn Gate

330 High Holborn

London WC1V 7BA

Telephone: +44 (0) 20 7430 0850

Fax: +44 (0) 20 7061 3390

E-mail: communications@hda-online.org.uk

Website: http://www.hda-online.org.uk

For Wales:

National Assembly for Wales

Cathays Park

Cardiff CF10 3NQ

Telephone: +44 (029) 2082 5111

Health Promotion Library,

Telephone: 029 2068 1245

E-mail: hplibrary@wales.gsi.gov.uk

Website: http://www.hpw.wales.gov.uk

For Scotland:

NHS Health Scotland

Woodburn House

Canaan Lane

Edinburgh EH10 4SG

Telephone: 0131 536 5500

Textphone: 0131 536 5503

Fax: 0131 536 5501

E-mail: public_affairs@hebs.scot.nhs.uk

publications@hebs.scot.nhs.uk

library.enquiries@hebs.scot.nhs.uk

Website: http://www.healthscotland.com

Note: These details continue to operate until the merger with PHIS is complete.

For Northern Ireland:

Health Promotion Agency for Northern Ireland

18 Ormeau Avenue

Belfast BT2 8HS

Telephone: +44 (0) 28 9031 1611

Fax: +44 (0) 28 9031 1711

E-mail: info@hpani.org.uk

Website: http://www.healthpromotionagency.org.uk

AN INTERNATIONAL LOOK AT HEALTH EDUCATION/ PROMOTION

This section provides a glimpse into some aspects of health and its promotion internationally. It is not intended as a thorough account of the situation in any of the countries mentioned, but as a sampler to illustrate a few interesting points about international health issues and how health and its promotion compare across different parts of the world.

Canada

In Canada, the national (federal) department responsible for health is Health Canada/Santé Canada. On its website, its activity is described in this way:

> In partnership with provincial and territorial governments, Health Canada provides national leadership to develop health policy, enforce health regulations, promote disease prevention and enhance healthy living for all Canadians. Health Canada ensures that health services are available and accessible to First Nations and Inuit communities. It also works closely with other federal departments, agencies and health stakeholders to reduce health and safety risks to Canadians.
> (Health Canada 2002a)

Health Canada's stated mission is 'To help the people of Canada maintain and improve their health', and it seeks to fulfil this by:

- Preventing and reducing risks to individual health and the overall environment

- Promoting healthier lifestyles

- Ensuring high-quality health services that are efficient and accessible

- Integrating renewal of the health care system with longer-term plans in the areas of prevention, health promotion and protection

- Reducing health inequalities in Canadian society; and

- Providing health information to help Canadians make informed decisions.
  (Health Canada 2003a)

A number of priority issues for health promotion and education are evident in the Health Canada website. General issues include the health of aboriginal peoples, food and nutrition, physical activity, alcohol and drug abuse, family violence, mental health, safety, sexuality and smoking. Specific illness-related issues include Acquired Immune Deficiency Syndrome (AIDS), cancer, diabetes, cardiovascular disease, hepatitis, Severe Acute Respiratory Syndrome (SARS), sexually transmitted diseases, and West Nile virus.

As in most other developed countries, Canada's health agenda places emphasis on chronic diseases and their causes. For example, there have been many initiatives designed to tackle the problem of smoking, such as the second-hand smoke campaign re-launched in September 2003. A campaign with a longer history is the VITALITY programme, which focuses on healthy living, with the slogan, 'Eating well, being active and feeling good about yourself – that's VITALITY'. It also encompasses messages about smoking, suggesting that healthy living habits provide positive alternatives to smoking (Health Canada 2002b). Such campaigns seek to promote health and prevent illness.

Two of Canada's recent priority health issues – SARS and the West Nile virus – provide interesting examples of how health education and promotion needs can arise, sometimes suddenly and unexpectedly.

The West Nile virus was first isolated in Uganda in 1933 (National Institute of Allergy and Infectious Diseases 2003). Its first emergence in the western hemisphere was in the United States in autumn 1999, in New York City (Illinois Department of Public Health 2003). The first confirmed human case of the virus in Canada was identified in September 2002 in Ontario. Although Health Canada believed this virus represented only a minor danger to humans, it responded by providing information in its online site about the virus, its symptoms and how to minimize risk (Health Canada 2003b). Thus members of the public could gain access to sound information online.

SARS first emerged in China in November 2002, and the largest number of cases elsewhere in the world was in Canada, mostly in Ontario. This understandably engendered fear in the population, as SARS could be fatal, and again Health Canada provided information on its website (Health Canada 2003c).

These examples illustrate how health issues that would once have remained relatively localized can quickly become international issues in today's world of rapid and frequent long-distance travel. The availability of information on the Health Canada website also illustrates how up-to-date technology can offer health teachers a useful way to disseminate information to the public.

Australia

In Australia, the Department of Health and Ageing has responsibility for health education and promotion. In 2002 the Department published seven national health priority areas: asthma, cancer control, cardiovascular health, diabetes mellitus, injury prevention and control, mental health, and arthritis and musculoskeletal conditions (Commonwealth Department of Health and Ageing 2003a). The Department works in collaboration with Australia's Territory governments on these priorities.

A particular form of cancer that has received special attention in Australia is skin cancer, which is the most common form of cancer there and is the cause of a significant level of mortality and morbidity (Livingstone et al 2001). It is believed that exposure to sun in childhood and adolescence is an important factor contributing to the development of skin cancer, and so health educators in Australia have given special attention to programmes that target school students and their parents.

In pursuing this and other health priorities, the Department of Health and Ageing sponsors a range of health promotion campaigns. One example is the annual Rock Eisteddfod Challenge. It offers secondary school students the opportunity to participate in dance and drama performances in front of live audiences. It has been shown to have popular appeal, and leads to a high level of recall of health messages. In 2003 this campaign included television specials promoting the National Alcohol Campaign message: 'Drinking – Where are your choices taking you?' (Commonwealth Department of Health and Ageing 2003b).

Another example is the Croc Festivals, which have been running since 1998. They are directed at primary and secondary school students living in remote and rural parts of Australia. Daytime activities focus on health, sports, role-modelling and performance art, among other things. They are primarily indigenous events, but other students participate as well. In evaluations, these Festivals have been shown to be successful in raising students' awareness of health messages in a form of communication that is appealing to them (Commonwealth Department of Health and Ageing 2003b).

The two examples above illustrate the variety of forms health teaching can take, and how it can be associated with various aspects of personal growth as well as entertainment.

South Africa

It is clear from South Africa's Department of Health website that some health issues that take priority in that country are quite different from those in countries like the UK, Canada and Australia. For example, malaria, cholera and tuberculosis are among the issues that appear on the website as having high priority. Not everything is different, however: tobacco also appears as a priority issue. Some issues that are nominally the same are very different in their impact, one of the most obvious being HIV/AIDS. In the UK, Canada and Australia, HIV/AIDS is indeed a health concern and the object of health teaching, but the difference in the magnitude of the health problem in South Africa is enormous. In 2001, for example, there were 379 deaths from HIV/AIDS in the UK; in South Africa, there were estimated to be 360,000 deaths from AIDS in that year (AVERT 2003). A health issue of this magnitude has a multitude of effects on the society. For example, it leaves orphaned children, many of whom are HIV-positive themselves, and it affects people of working age, including health workers. Thus it represents a major health challenge that cannot be ignored by the government and health agencies.

HIV/AIDS in poor and developing countries has been in the news recently in relation to the availability of drug treatment. For example, an article in The Guardian newspaper in the UK in October 2003 reported an agreement made with drug companies by former US president Bill Clinton. This agreement should make it possible to get cheaper drugs to the large numbers of people with HIV/AIDS in South Africa and other countries in similar circumstances. Alongside such treatment initiatives, however, there remains a challenging job for health organizations and health teachers.

The National AIDS Unit of the Department of Health (Department of Health [South Africa] 2003) has particular responsibility for addressing this health problem. Its mission is:

> To reduce the transmission of STDs [sexually transmitted diseases] (including HIV infection) and provide appropriate treatment, care and support for those infected and affected, through collaborative efforts within all levels of government, using the NACOSA national AIDS Plan as the terms of reference.

One particular way in which South Africa has been tackling this challenge is through its Youth Programme, which includes Life-Skills Programs in primary and secondary schools, and the Youth AIDS Program (Department of Health [South Africa] 2003).

Another project is the 'loveLife train'. This is run as part of an initiative supported by the Henry J. Kaiser Family Foundation and carried out in partnership with the South African government and Spoornet, which is the provider of rail freight in South Africa. (Additional support for this initiative comes from the Bill and Melinda Gates Foundation, the Nelson Mandela Foundation and the Anglo-American Corporation). The 'loveLife' initiative is 'a bold and ambitious attempt to reduce HIV infection among South African adolescents by promoting sexual health and healthy futures for young people' (KFF 2003). The 'loveLife train' is 'a community project [that] travels from station to station stopping for six days at each station throughout the country ... to provide free legal advice, HIV/AIDS awareness and life skills' (Health Systems Trust 2003).

The above examples taken from three countries around the world demonstrate the wide and varied range of challenges that can face those whose job it is to 'teach for health'. They also illustrate what might be called the 'connectedness' of international health issues and health promotion. Although there are some wide differences between the issues in various countries, both health problems (such as HIV and SARS) and measures to promote and improve health (such as the activities of benevolent foundations) can cross national boundaries.

NURSES AS HEALTH TEACHERS

Nurses have taught people about health since the establishment of the profession. In the early days the teaching reflected the general concern about sanitation and living conditions. In her *Notes on Nursing* (1859), Florence Nightingale emphasized that ill health was the result of want of whitewashing and ventilation, as well as careless diet and dress. She proposed that the nurse should act as educator in these areas.

Perhaps one of the best-known and most widely accepted statements on nursing is that prepared by Virginia Henderson (1960) for the International Council of Nurses in 1961. It describes the unique function of the nurse as assisting the individual, sick or well, in health-related activities which he would perform unaided if he had the necessary strength, will or knowledge. That the nurse has a health education role is implicit in this statement. Moreover, Henderson indicates something of the extent and nature of the role: the nurse assists the person to gain motivation as well as knowledge and skills and she directs her energies to the well population and to the sick.

Nurses, like all other health educators, have a changing role in health education. Clearly, the nature of health education activity considered to be suitable will depend on the environment in which nursing takes place and there will be many different interpretations of the term. Some nurses have described health teaching as a nursing tool, to be used to promote spiritual, mental and physical health. Others have gone further and suggested that the nature of nursing is such that teaching is of the very essence of nursing. Reviews of how the nurse's education role is perceived were provided in the early 1980s by

Redman (1980) and Cohen (1981). These reviews indicated that most nurses accepted that they had a health education role, though there was confusion over the extent and nature of the activity required, and uncertainty about how the nurse's role complemented or differed from that of the doctor. In a survey of senior nurses in England a decade later, Latter et al (1992) found that health education was generally perceived to be a part of nursing practice in acute hospital wards, and numerous articles in the 1990s indicate an acceptance that health education is part of the nurse's role.

It is relevant to note the introduction of new diploma level courses (referred to at the time as 'Project 2000' courses) throughout the UK during the early 1990s. These programmes place strong emphasis on health rather than focusing primarily on illness as previous programmes did. However, it has also been found that students and nurses are often unclear about the meanings of the terms 'health education' and 'health promotion', and the difference between them (Davis 1995; MacLeod Clark et al 1998).

The nurse's role as health teacher may arise as part of the usual process of nurse-patient interaction: the nurse reads cues which indicate the patient's readiness to learn and responds to these by seizing or creating the opportunity for teaching (Narrow 1979; Redman 1980). Thus health education by nurses may be individually tailored to needs, and delivery can be instantaneous. This view suggests that the skilled nurse will identify gaps in the patient's knowledge, sense how much information he wants, judge whether the patient is comfortable or relaxed enough to take in the information, and gear the language and explanation to such factors as the patient's social class, education and experience, as well as psychological and emotional readiness. The nurse will also, as appropriate, make use of visual aids or written materials to augment verbal explanations.

The model of health education proposed is an educational one and fits well into a nursing process framework. Nurses exercise their professional skills in assessing people's teaching needs, in planning and conducting appropriate teaching, and in evaluating the outcome of the teaching plan. In a statement about the patient education skills required by registered nurses, the General Nursing Council for Scotland (1980) noted that the nurse needed to:

- identify the learning needs of patients and relatives

- identify the learning opportunities available for individuals and/or groups in the clinical setting

- select and use suitable teaching methods and materials

- develop patient education within (a given) care setting

- evaluate patient education programmes at a level which will allow for improvement of personal performance as a health teacher.

This list reflects the importance and complexity of the modern health education role in nursing, and implies endorsement of the educational model.

A similar endorsement was evident in a 1983 publication of the Scottish National Nursing and Midwifery Consultative Committee (SHHD 1983) which proposed that health education should be applied within the process of nursing to assist the individual to identify and take informed decisions about his health potential and health-related behaviour. This report, while it proposed that nurses should adopt a systematic approach to the planning and implementing of health education, counselled that such planning need not imply inflexibility nor the imposition of professional values.

The concept of consumer participation was evident in the movement which has been called self-care (Levin et al 1977). This concept assumes that the individual's integrity in making health decisions, and his ability to perform on his own behalf, take precedence over professional values. Self-care, therefore, means that patients may be involved in procedures previously carried out by medical and nursing staff and in taking responsibility for certain decisions about care. Self-care means more than self-treatment, however. Health maintenance, disease prevention, self-diagnosis, self-medication and participation in professional care have also been identified as possible roles for the individual to adopt. Perhaps the most challenging aspect of the self-care concept is that it acknowledges that evaluation of care is based on what the individual sees as relevant, not on professional criteria of effectiveness.

Active participation by patients in their care requires a balancing of professional and patient goals, with emphasis on the development of professional-lay relationships and mutual respect, and the avoidance of attempts at domination by professionals. In health education it means accepting that the health professional does not always know best. There is obvious scope within traditional nursing care for the development of teaching geared to participation. Patients may learn on an individual basis as they participate in their care. Such learning may be supplemented by group sessions and use of visual aids or written materials. There are also important learning opportunities inherent in participating in decision-making and undertaking self-treatment under agreed levels of professional supervision.

The appropriateness of such shifts in the emphases in nursing care – from control in the hands of the professional towards control in the hands of the patient or client, from care-giving to teaching and enabling – has been accelerating in recent years due to the nature of changes taking place in the health service and in nursing. There has been a deliberate move away from hospital care towards care in the community, from focusing on illness to focusing on health. Health education is vital to the success of such change.

Macleod Clark and Webb said in 1985, 'Health education is one of the most important and challenging facets of a nurse's role. Paradoxically it is also a facet which is poorly understood and greatly undervalued' (p. 210). In the intervening years, the second statement in this quotation has probably become less true. One indication of this can be found in the curricula of the diploma and undergraduate nursing programmes. The 'Project 2000' document which led to the development of the higher education diploma programmes highlighted the importance of this approach to nursing:

> ... any CFP [Common Foundation Programme] must be embedded in health not in illness. It must be closely allied to the stated goals of the NHS in relation to the various care groups, namely to restore health, to teach self-care, to promote independent living as far as this is possible, and to respect the values and desires of the individual patient or client. This means that from the very start therefore, the student must learn about normal living, about the range of normal reactions to stress, about coping and about the importance of support. The student must learn that

care is not always 'doing for' or 'doing to', and that the skills do not lie solely in practical activities but are based on a wider concept of health and healing. (UKCC 1986 p. 46)

Curriculum content was to be divided into seven subject themes, and one of these was 'health education and promotion'.

More recent evidence of this shift in emphasis can be seen in the 2001 Scottish strategy document for nursing and midwifery, *Caring for Scotland*, which gives a prominent place to 'the change in NHS culture from one of illness and treatment, to one of health promotion and illness prevention' and 'encouraging individuals to take responsibility for improving their health' (SEHD 2001 p. 7).

While the educational model of health education may appear best to fit the demands described above, there may be a case for considering that all five approaches outlined earlier are relevant for the nurse as health teacher. A report on the health education in-service training needs of nurses (SHEG 1983) recorded the idea that no single model of health education may meet the variety of situations in which nurses operate, and this may be even more true now. If people are to take more control of their own health, then perhaps the community development and political action models have much to offer. It might be argued, however, that the educational model can provide a starting point, a foundation upon which to build, and that it can be used in conjunction with any of the other four models. The discussion in the next section addresses this matter further.

TEACHING FOR HEALTH

Although health education varies in form and philosophy, and nursing practice in health education will be similarly varied, this text has been entitled *Teaching for Health* on the assumption that the student of nursing (or midwifery, or any of the allied health professions) is most likely to experience and practise health education based on an educational model. The educational model assumes that health behaviour is the result of learning and that it therefore can be influenced by an educational process in which the nurse or other professional assumes the role of teacher or enabler and the patient or client accepts the role of learner. In this text the process has been labelled 'teaching for health'.

Some nurses find it difficult to distinguish the teaching aspect of their work. Much of nursing is directed at assisting adaptation to the circumstances surrounding health and illness. Since learning is an essential part of adapting, it can be argued that all nursing is teaching. At the other extreme, some nurses may have a view of teaching based upon earlier schooldays and see it as a 'talk and chalk' experience.

This text assumes that health teaching is an integral part of nursing and that it should be executed as a purposeful activity, using interactive teaching strategies which involve the learner in planning and evaluating his learning wherever possible.

In teaching for health, the nurse may help to identify and solve health-related problems by:

- informing
- advising
- helping with the acquisition of skills
- assisting with the process of clarifying beliefs, feelings and values
- enabling the adaptation of lifestyle
- promoting change in the structures and organizations which influence health status
- providing a model of values and behaviour related to health.

The last may present the individual nurse with a particularly difficult challenge. Most people feel uncomfortable being viewed as good examples, exemplary role models. There is no easy answer to this. Patients and clients observe the nurse's behaviour and learn from it regardless of the nurse's intentions. This does offer an element of responsibility to the individual nurse – what Gordon has referred to as patients' or clients' 'expectations of a healthy example' (1999 p. 101) – which implies a certain ethical quandary in relation to nurses' own rights to autonomy. Perhaps what can be said is that each nurse has the same right as any other person to be healthy and that her or his decisions about health should not be considered only in the light of the impact upon patients or clients.

All nurses have the right to decide for themselves how they will give expression to their health teaching function. The approach taken will no doubt reflect each individual's philosophy of nursing and of life, as well as beliefs about the nature and purpose of health education. The following chapter will address some detailed aspects of the teaching and learning process.

REFERENCES

Anon 1881 Health lectures for the people. MacNiven and Wallace, Edinburgh.

AVERT 2003 HIV & AIDS statistics. AVERT.org, Horsham, West Sussex.

Blaxter M 1990 Health & lifestyles. Tavistock/Routledge, London.

Clark D, McKeon A, Sutton M, Wood R 2004 Healthy Life Expectancy in Scotland. ISD Scotland, Edinburgh.

Cohen S A 1981 Patient education: a review of the literature. Journal of Advanced Nursing (6): 11-16.

Commonwealth Department of Health and Ageing 2003a National Health Priorities & Quality. http://www.health.gov.au/pq/index.htm Accessed October 20, 2003.

Commonwealth Department of Health and Ageing 2003b Campaigns and events calendar. http://www.health.gov.au/campaigns.htm Accessed October 20, 2003.

Daley A 1959 The central council for health education the first twenty-five years 1927-52. The Health Education Journal 17(1): 24-35.

Davis S 1995 An investigation into nurses' understanding of health education and health promotion within a neuro-rehabilitation setting. Journal of Advanced Nursing 21(5): 951-959.

Department of Health 1992 The Health of the Nation: a strategy for health in England. Cm 1986. HMSO, London.

Department of Health 1999/2003 Saving Lives: Our Healthier Nation website: http://www.ohn.gov.uk/ Accessed April 4, 2003.

Department of Health [South Africa] 2003 Issues – National AIDS Unit, Department of Health. http://www.doh.gov.za/issues/index.html Accessed October 24, 2003.

Department of Health and Social Security 1980 Inequalities in health: report of a research working group (The Black Report). DHSS, London.

Department of Health and Personal Social Services 1993 A regional strategy for the Northern Ireland health & personal social services 1992-1997. Northern Ireland

Department of Health and Personal Social Services.

Felvus J 1991 Lessons in protocol. The Health Service Journal. 100(5237) (7 February): 20-21.

Ewles L, Simnett I 1999 Promoting Health, 4th Edition. Balliere Tindall/Royal College of Nursing, London.

Guardian (2003) Clinton deal to get AIDS drugs to world's poor. Guardian, Friday October 24 2003.

General Nursing Council for Scotland 1980 Guidelines on health education. General Nursing Council, Edinburgh.

Gordon MF 1999 The Representation of Professional Identity: The Health Promotion Discourse of Hospital Nurses. Unpublished PhD thesis, University of Aberdeen.

Health Canada/Santé Canada 2002a Health Canada Online – What we do. http://www.hc-sc.gc.ca/english/about/about.html Accessed October 20, 2003.

Health Canada/Santé Canada 2002b Health Canada Online – VITALITY: a positive approach to healthy living. http://www.hc-sc.gc.ca/phfb-dgpsa/onpp-bppn/leaders_approach_e.html Accessed October 20, 2003.

Health Canada/Santé Canada 2003a Health Canada Online – 2003-2004 Estimates Part III – Report on plans and priorities. http://www.tbs-sct.gc.ca/est-pre/20032004/hlth-sant/hlth-santr34_e.asp Accessed October 20, 2003.

Health Canada/Santé Canada 2003b Health Canada Online – West Nile virus. http://www.hc-sc.gc.ca/english/westnile/index.html Accessed October 20, 2003.

Health Canada/Santé Canada 2003c Health Canada Online – Learning from SARS – Renewal of public health in Canada, Executive Summary. http://www.hc-sc.gc.ca/english/protection/warnings/sars/learning/EngSe30_exec.htm Accessed October 20, 2003.

Health Education Authority 1993 Operational Plan. HEA, London.

Health Education Authority July 1994 Information sheet. HEA, London.

Health Promotion Agency 2003 Health Promotion Agency home page, Health Promotion Agency website: http://www.healthpromotionagency.org.uk/ Accessed June 7, 2003.

Health Promotion Authority for Wales (HPA) 1990a Health for all in Wales, Part A:

Strategies for action. HPA, Cardiff.

Health Promotion Authority for Wales (HPA) 1990b Health for all in Wales, Part B: Health Promotion challenges for the 1990s. HPA, Cardiff.

Health Promotion Authority for Wales (HPA) 1990c Health for all in Wales, Part C: Strategic directions for the Health Promotion Authority. HPA, Cardiff.

Health Promotion Division 2001 Promoting health and well being: Implementing the national health promotion strategy. The National Assembly for Wales, Cardiff.

Health Systems Trust 2003 Spoornet puts love train back on the rails for another year. Health Systems Trust, Durban. http://new.hst.org.za/news/index.php/20030220/ Accessed October 24, 2003.

Henderson V 1960 Basic principles of nursing care. International Council of Nurses. Basle, Switzerland (reprinted 1970).

Illich I 1971 Deschooling society. Calder and Boyars, London.

Illich I 1974 Medical nemesis: the expropriation of health. Calder and Boyars, London.

Illinois Department of Public Health 2003 West Nile Virus. IDPH Online http://www.idph.state.il.us/envhealth/wnf.htm Accessed October 20, 2003.

Jones L, Naidoo J 2000 Theories and Models in Health Promotion. In J Katz, A Peberdy & J Douglas (Eds), Promoting Health – Knowledge and Practice, 2nd Edition. The Open University/Palgrave, Oxford. Pages 80-94.

Kennedy I 1981 The unmasking of medicine. George Allen & Unwin, London.

Kickbush I 1983 Introducing the regional programme on health education and lifestyles. Community Medicine 5(1): 59-62.

Latter S, Macleod Clark J, Wilson Barnett J, Maben J 1992 Health education in nursing: perceptions of practice in acute settings. Journal of Advanced Nursing 17(1): 164-172.

Levin LS, Katz AH, Holst E 1977 Self-care: lay initiatives in health. Croom Helm, London.

Livingstone PM, White VM, Ugoni AM, Borland R 2001 Knowledge, attitudes and self-care practices related to sun protection among secondary students in Australia. Health Education Research 16(3): 269-278.

Mackintosh N 1996 Promoting health: an issue for nursing. Quay Books, Dinton.

Macleod Clark J, Maben J, Jones K 1998 Health promotion: perceptions of Project 2000 educated nurses. Health Education Research 13(2): 185-196.

Macleod Clark J, Webb P 1985 Health

education–a basis for professional nursing practice. Nurse Education Today 5: 210-214.

McKenna F 2003 Background information on Northern Ireland society – population and vital statistics. CAIN Web Service. http://www.cain.ulst.ac.uk/ni/popul.htm Accessed September 10, 2003.

McKeown T 1976 The role of medicine: dream mirage or nemesis. Rock Carling Lecture, Nuffield Provincial Hospitals Trust, London.

Ministry of Health 1964 Report of a joint committee of the Central and Scottish Health Services Councils on health education (The Cohen Report). HMSO, London.

Narrow BW 1979 Patient teaching in nursing practice: a patient and family centred approach. John Wiley, New York.

National Institute of Allergy and Infectious Diseases 2003 NIAID research on West Nile virus. National Institutes of Health, Bethesda Maryland. http://www.niaid.nih.gov/factsheets/westnile.htm Accessed October 20, 2003

Nightingale F 1859 Notes on nursing. Harrison and Sons, Reprinted 1980 Churchill Livingstone, Edinburgh.

Norton L 1998 Health promotion and health education: what role should the nurse adopt in practice? Journal of Advanced Nursing 28(6): 1269-1275.

Phillips L 1995 Chattanooga Creek: case study of the public health nursing role in environmental health. Public Health Nursing 12(5): 335-40.

Pisharoti KA 1975 Guide to the integration of health education in environmental health programmes. WHO offset publication No 20, WHO, Geneva.

Rawson D, Grigg C 1988 Purpose & practice in health education. South Bank Polytechnic/HEA, London.

Redman BK 1980 The process of patient teaching in nursing, 4th edn. Mosby, St Louis.

Scottish Executive Department of Health [SEHD] 2001 Caring for Scotland: The Strategy for Nursing and Midwifery in Scotland. Edinburgh: Scottish Executive.

Scottish Health Education Group 1983 Health education in-service training needs of district nurses health visitors and midwives. SHEG, Edinburgh.

Scottish Home and Health Department 1983 Health education and nursing. A report by the national nursing and midwifery consultative committee. SHHD, Edinburgh.

Scottish Home and Health Department 1989 A review of health education in Scotland. Touche Ross Management Consultants, SHHD, Edinburgh.

Scottish Office Home and Health Department 1991 Health education in Scotland: a national policy statement. SOHHD, Edinburgh.

Scottish Office Home and Health Department 1992 Scotland's health: a challenge to us all. SOHHD, Edinburgh.

Scottish Office Home and Health Department [no date] Scotland's health: a challenge to you. SOHHD, Edinburgh.

Simonds SK 1977 Health education today: issues and challenges. The Journal of School Health December: 584-593.

Smithies J, Webster G 1998 Community Involvement in Health: From Passive Recipients to Active Participants. Ashgate, Aldershot.

Smout TC 1986 A century of the Scottish people 1830-1950. Fontana, London.

Statutory Instruments 1987 No 6. National Health Service, England and Wales. The Health Education Authority (Establishment and Constitution) Order 1987. HMSO, London.

Thompson IE 1983 Theoretical models of health education. In: Scottish Health Education Group. Health education in-service training needs of district nurses health visitors and midwives. Scottish Health Education Group, Edinburgh.

Thomson D 1965 England in the twentieth century (1914-63). Penguin, Harmondsworth.

Tones BK 1977 The role of the community health education specialist in the delivery of health care. The Health Education Journal 36(4): 106-133.

Tones BK 1979 Socialisation health career and the health education of the school child. Journal of the Institute of Health Education 17(1): 22-28.

United Kingdom Central Council for Nursing, Midwifery and Health Visiting (UKCC) 1986 Project 2000: a new preparation for practice. UKCC, London.

Vuori H 1980 The medical model and the objectives of health education. International Journal of Health Education (19): 12-18.

Welsh Health Planning Forum 1989 Strategic intent and direction for the NHS in Wales. Welsh Office NHS Directorate.

Whitehead D 2001 Health eduation, behavioural change and social psychology: nursing's contribution to health promotion? Journal of Advanced Nursing 34(6): 822-832.

Whitehead M 1987 The health divide:

inequalities in health in the 1980s. Health Education Council, London.

Wilson M 1975 Health is for people. Dartmann Longman Todd. London.

World Health Organization 1947 Constitution of the WHO. Chronicle of the WHO 1(3): 1.

World Health Organization 1954 Expert committee on health education of the public: first report. Technical Report Series No 89 WHO, Geneva.

World Health Organization 1958 Report of an expert committee on training of health personnel in health education of the public. Technical Report Series No 156. WHO, Geneva.

World Health Organization 1969 Report of an expert committee on planning and evaluation of health education services. Technical Report Series No 409. WHO, Geneva.

World Health Organization 1978 Primary health care. Report of the International Conference on Primary Health Care. Alma Ata USSR 6-12 September. WHO, Geneva.

World Health Organization 1981 Regional programme in health education and lifestyles. Regional Committee for Europe Thirty-first session, Berlin 15-19 September EUR/RC31/10. WHO, Copenhagen.

World Health Organization 1986 Ottawa Charter for health promotion. WHO, Geneva.

Wohl AS 1983 Endangered lives: public health in Victorian Britain. Methuen, London.

3 Learning about health

IDEAS ABOUT LEARNING AND TEACHING

There is an essential relationship between teaching and learning, and it could be argued that although it is possible to learn without being taught, it is not possible to teach without learning taking place. That is, if no learning has occurred, then teaching did not occur either. Telling might have occurred, but not teaching. So it is important for the health professional who embarks upon teaching to give careful thought to what learning is and how it occurs.

Defining teaching

The term 'teaching' encompasses a variety of activities. These include giving information or advice, counselling and helping people clarify their thinking, express their feelings, identify options or develop new skills. Teaching may be defined as the process of helping or enabling another person to learn. Some teaching is done deliberately according to a plan: school teachers teach spelling, driving instructors teach how to control the car, midwives teach about breast-feeding, and so on. Other teaching may not be deliberate: parents may teach their children how to smoke, school teachers may convince children that mathematics is important only for boys, doctors may teach patients to expect prescriptions. So there is unintended as well as intended teaching.

Defining learning

Learning is a basic human activity, essential to survival. Young children have to be protected from heat, cold, water, heights and road traffic until they have learned about the dangers. The ability to learn helps us avoid danger, communicate with others, adapt to changed circumstances, earn a living, or enjoy the finer aspects of any art form. Learning may be conscious or unconscious, easy or difficult, painful or pleasant. Much of the time learning is taken for granted. But what is involved in learning?

Psychologists say learning is demonstrated by a change in behaviour. At two years old, a child may run into the street if the garden gate is left open. Within a few years he will usually have acquired the habit of stopping by the kerb to check for oncoming traffic. It is concluded that he has learned to cross the road safely. That learning has taken place is inferred because his behaviour has changed. Changed behaviour confirms learning. But what happened within the child to bring about the learning? From everyday observation we may reach a number of conclusions as to what may have gone on:

- He may have learned from experience – perhaps he stepped out and got hurt.

- He may have learned because something frightened him – perhaps he saw someone knocked down by a car.

- He may have come to an understanding of danger and an acceptance of the need to avoid it, by having it explained and being told stories or shown pictures.

These are reasonable explanations, as far as they go. They illustrate that there may be three ways to learn: through doing, feeling and thinking. The child's behaviour has changed because he now has a concept of danger related to motor cars and he has been motivated to avoid the danger. In this case the motivation may have come from fear, from experience or from an inculcated sense of responsibility. Another possible explanation would be that the avoidance of danger is an instinctual reaction. Human learning is complex. Learning theorists have provided a variety of explanations of how learning takes place and what motivates it. These will be considered in some detail later in this chapter.

The teaching–learning process

The process of teaching and learning is an interactive one: both learner and teacher have to be actively involved. Factors in the learner, the teacher and the teaching environment all create the teaching situation and influence the outcome of teaching and learning. The responsibility for what goes on in teaching and learning does not lie exclusively with either of the partners in the process, nor can it either depend solely upon or be divorced from the environment in which it occurs. Figure 3.1 illustrates some of the interrelated factors in teaching and learning.

Health teaching should be designed to meet the needs of the learner and encourage accountability in both teacher and learner. A systematic but flexible approach is preferable to a reliance on incidental teaching. The use of a planned procedure helps both participants in the teaching–learning process to identify and focus on specific learning needs, to plan how to meet those needs, to put the plans into action and then to evaluate whether learning occurred.

Using a planned process for health teaching means focusing on what is needed. Ideally, the learner should participate at all stages to help identify

FIGURE 3.1   *Factors in the teaching–learning situation*

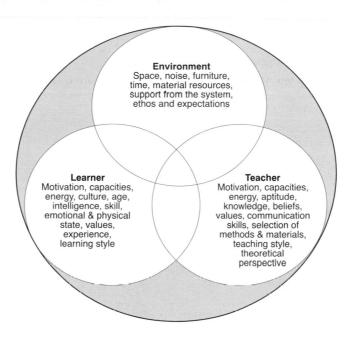

what knowledge, attitudes and behaviours he needs to acquire in relation to his health status. A systematic approach to teaching and learning contributes to comprehensive assessment and renders accountability possible by promoting the prediction of success. It may also enhance efficiency in health care settings but this should not be the prime factor in utilizing a planned process. Cost effectiveness as the main motivator for health teaching is in conflict with some values associated with concepts such as prevention and promotion. Cost-related goals are more usually related to institutions and professions, not client satisfaction or participation.

Problem-solving approaches to teaching and learning are characterized by attempts to ensure objectivity, rationality and applicability. Though these are desirable elements in any programme of care, they present certain dangers in health teaching, since they may encourage a mechanistic approach to assessing, planning and implementing teaching. Routine, even rigid, deployment of the health teaching process may be avoided by encouraging each patient or client to participate to the fullest degree possible in assessing learning needs and planning how the learning will take place. The unique nature of each individual and the nurse's idiosyncratic way of viewing an individual's needs force nurses to consider a world view which may differ radically from their own. Thus each individual undergoing surgery, for instance, will have some common and some unique preoperative learning needs. Health teaching as a planned process facilitates knowledgeable self-care, and promotes and accepts the responsibility of individuals for their own health decisions.

THEORETICAL CONSIDERATIONS RELEVANT TO LEARNING

Learning theories

Most learning theories have been derived from experiments under laboratory-type conditions, sometimes with animals rather than humans, and they therefore need to be applied with caution to everyday life. Nonetheless, learning theories can help to interpret people's behaviour while learning and also can suggest solutions to some learning problems. Thus it is useful for the health teacher to have a basic understanding of major learning theories.

Behaviourist (associative) learning theories

According to these theories, learning can be explained as a connection, made by the learner, between a stimulus and a response. The process by which such a connection is made has been labelled 'conditioning'. Two types of conditioning have been distinguished: classical and operant (or instrumental).

Classical conditioning was first described by Pavlov who noted that dogs salivated in response to the sight of food. He labelled this 'unconditioned response', because training was not needed to elicit it. He experimented by sounding a bell regularly before the dog's food was served and discovered that the dog could be trained to salivate upon hearing the bell, even when no food was given. This he labelled 'conditioned response' (Romiszowski 1988).

Operant conditioning is also an explanation of trained response but in this case the subject of the experiment 'operates' the environment in such a way as to receive a reward. Classic examples of operant conditioning are the experiments carried out by the psychologist Skinner who showed that pigeons exploring their boxes could be trained to operate a lever to deliver food. In this case the food was the reward for, or 'reinforcer' of, the learning. In a series of experiments, Skinner demonstrated that learning could be induced by administering carefully planned rewards according to a plan he referred to as a schedule of reinforcements (Skinner 1953).

An important feature of the behaviourist theories is that they view the learner as being largely passive as far as learning itself goes. The learner is merely adopting certain responses according to his experience of the stimulus and its effects.

Useful points that can be taken from the behaviourist school of thinking (Hartley 1998) are:

- Activity is important.
- Repetition, generalization and discrimination are important notions.
- Reinforcement is the cardinal motivator.
- Learning is helped when objectives are clear.

Cognitive learning theories

These theories, on the other hand, stress the importance of the learner's own thinking or cognitive processes. They offer explanations for more complex

FIGURE 3.2   *Combining Bruner's and Ausubel's views of effective learning*

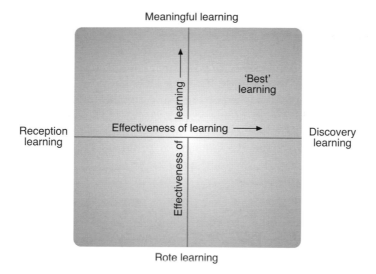

forms of learning, such as the learning involved when human beings solve problems or process information. Central to cognitive learning theories is the idea of perception, which is concerned with how human beings make sense of the world around them. Perception is the process which varies when individuals look at the same object but see it differently. In other words, the response to the stimulus (the object viewed) may differ because the individual's personal make-up and previous experience will influence how he perceives the object. Experiments have shown that both cultural expectations and past experience influence how individuals perceive things.

Among the cognitive theorists, two important names are those of Bruner and Ausubel. Bruner (1960, 1964) highlighted the value of what he termed 'discovery learning', as distinguished from 'reception learning'. He believed that students should be encouraged to be inquisitive rather than being trained to accept knowledge that was merely passed on to them. Ausubel emphasized the need for learning to be meaningful rather than rote (Ausubel 1968; Ausubel et al 1978). As learning is acquired, the result is unique, being the product of the interaction between incoming information and the learner's own cognitive structure. These views of learning are illustrated schematically in Figure 3.2. It can be seen that according to these theories, the most effective learning is that which could be plotted in the upper right quadrant of the diagram.

A group of well-known early cognitive theorists were the Gestalt psychologists (e.g. Köhler 1929, Koffka 1935), who gave to the German word 'Gestalt', which means patterns, a new meaning in psychology when they used it to refer to 'wholes'. They suggested that breaking human behaviour down into small pieces was potentially distorting and that the true meaning of the behaviour was thus likely to be lost. Gestalt theorists recognized that the whole is sometimes greater than the sum of its parts, and that people see and interpret things as wholes rather than by considering the bits and pieces that go to make up the picture. Gestalt psychologists were concerned to consider how the individual's perception of a situation would influence the way he responded to any given stimulus. They demonstrated the tendency for people to make sense of things by grouping items or seeing patterns.

An important idea from Gestalt psychology is that of insight. There are times when learning seems to happen all at once; the individual suddenly feels that he now understands. This has been described as the 'aha!' reaction. Most people can recall such moments, and sometimes it is even possible to observe them happening in other people. Having insight means seeing relationships which make the previously meaningless make sense. Gaining insight allows the individual to solve the immediate problem and apply what he or she has learned to similar situations in the future.

Useful principles that can be drawn from the cognitive theorists (Hartley 1998) include:

- Instruction should be well organized.
- Instruction should be clearly structured.
- The perceptual features of the task are important.
- Prior knowledge is important.
- Differences between individuals are important.
- Cognitive feedback gives information to learners about their success or failure concerning the task at hand.

Other theories

There are several other theories of learning that do not quite fit into the two types discussed above. Two that are particularly worth noting could be seen as extensions of the cognitive theories, and are, in fact, sometimes placed within that category.

The first of these types is sometimes given the label 'humanist'. One of the best known theorists in this category is Carl Rogers. His views of learning acknowledge the feelings component, along with the thinking and perceiving components. For Rogers, the individuality of the learner is important, and the learner must be given freedom of self-expression and the teacher's unqualified regard for him or her as a person (Rogers & Freiberg 1994). Thus the learner is the centre of the learning process, and the process of learning takes precedence over the information to be learned: 'The only man who is educated is the man who has learned how to learn' (Rogers 1969 p. 103).

The second type of theory to be considered here, the constructivist view of learning, further develops some of the ideas of the cognitive theorists, especially Bruner, as well as those of Rogers. The core premise of constructivist theory is that people construct their own understanding and knowledge of the world through their experiences and reflection on those experiences (Funderstanding 1998-2001). For learning to be meaningful, the learning context must take account of the psychological, social, cultural and historical factors that affect the individual learner (Maslovaty & Kuzi 2002). Among constructivist theorists, Nisbet emphasizes the importance of 'metacognition', which is described as 'being aware of what one is doing, or being able to bring one's mental

TABLE 3.1	*Views of the learner in four categories of learning theory*

Type of theory	Assumptions about the learner's behaviour
Behaviourist or associative	The learner responds to a stimulus
Cognitive	The learner thinks and responds or acts
Humanist	The learner thinks, feels, believes, values, etc., and acts
Constructivist	The learner thinks, feels, believes, values, etc., integrates new perceptions with existing conceptual understandings, and acts, and is capable of understanding the processes of his or her own learning

processes under conscious scrutiny and thus more effectively under control' (Nisbet & Shucksmith 1986 p. 7). When the learner is successful in this, he or she is better able to transfer learning strategies from one situation to another.

The views of the learner encompassed by the types of theories discussed above are compared in Table 3.1. Each type of theory has something to offer, and the teacher of health should draw on them according to their relevance for different learning situations.

From a range of 'other theories' (other than behaviourist or cognitive), the following points for practice (Smith 1999) are relevant:

- Learning is in the relationships between people.

- Educators work so that people can become participants in communities of practice.

- There is an intimate connection between knowledge and activity.

Domains of learning

Learning theorists have described three domains of learning (see Figure 3.3):

- *The cognitive domain.* This refers to the acquisition of information, facts, explanations, and the ability to work with this knowledge. It entails skills such as recognition, recall, description, explanation, analysis and synthesis. Examples would include learning about the function of insulin, learning how smoking affects the lungs, learning what to expect after surgery, or learning the principles of a healthy diet.

- *The psychomotor domain.* This refers to the learning of skills of 'doing'. It entails the development of dexterity in carrying out physical or technical tasks. Examples would include learning how to give an insulin injection, learning post-mastectomy exercises, learning to cook, or learning how to apply a condom correctly.

- *The affective domain.* This refers to the learning of values, attitudes, beliefs or feelings. It entails a change in the person's orientation or perspective on a given issue, which means that the person learns to accept the value as well as the facts of the matter, and develops skill in judgement. Examples would include accepting the importance of taking one's epilepsy medication, accepting the need to avoid unprotected casual sexual activity, accepting the value of regular exercise, or accepting the validity of respect for individual dignity.

FIGURE 3.3   *Learning levels in the three domains of learning (From Bloom 1956, with permission of McGraw Hill Education)*

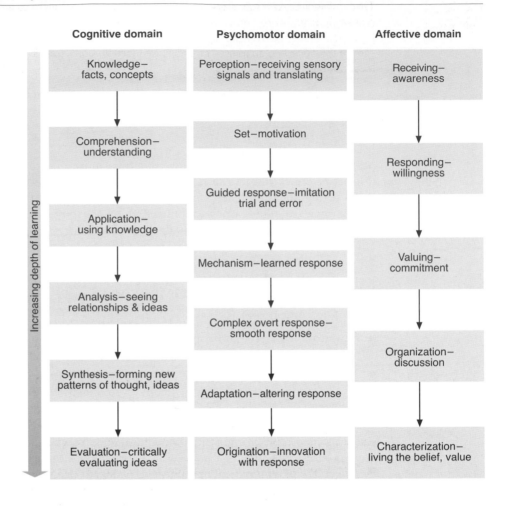

Much learning relates to more than one of the three domains. In the case of sexual health education, for example, the desired learning might entail learning the facts about sexually transmitted diseases (STDs), learning how to use a condom, and accepting the need either to avoid casual sexual activity or to use a condom. If an individual decides to indulge in casual sexual activity, has learned the facts about STDs, and knows how to use a condom but doesn't bother because 'It won't happen to me', then full learning has not taken place. The cognitive and psychomotor learning was achieved, but the failure in the affective domain makes that learning virtually worthless. Thus, when teaching is being planned, it is important for the planner to take account of the relevance of learning in all three domains.

ACTIVITY 3.1

Think of five important topics or areas of learning you have been involved in within the past week or so. For each one, identify which of the three domains of learning it involved. If you immediately place a learning experience within one domain, be sure to think about each of the other two domains – it may involve more than one, even if one seems the most obvious.

Levels of learning

It is generally acknowledged that there are different levels of learning, and that the process of learning may involve moving through a hierarchy. This implies that the learner proceeds from the concrete to the abstract or from lower level skills to higher level skills. Gagné (1974), in his discussion of the acquisition of intellectual skills, lists eight categories of learning beginning with the simplest, the development of involuntary behaviour through classical conditioning. He proposes that an individual has to proceed through each level successfully in order to be prepared to tackle the next level. After an initial period in which he merely recognizes and responds to stimuli, the learner will progress to more complex forms of learning such as verbal associations, differentiation of stimuli, concept formation and, finally, problem solving. One well-known classification of learning types and levels is Bloom's Taxonomy (Bloom 1956, Krathwohl et al 1964). Cognitive, affective and psychomotor learning levels proposed by Bloom and his colleagues are summarized in Figure 3.3.

As with the domains of learning, the health teacher needs to consider the level of learning that is needed for the task in hand. For example, does the person with a stoma have to be able to innovate in managing appliances, or will it be enough to follow mechanically the pattern set by the nursing staff in hospital? If she has to accomplish origination (see Figure 3.3), by what stage in the postoperative progress will this be a reasonable expectation – immediately prior to discharge, at the first outpatient appointment or within one year of surgery?

If the learning process is hierarchical, then this has implications for the teacher. It will be important to establish an appropriate starting point for the learner, and learners may need support in seeing how to build from one level of complexity to the next. In addition, teaching should usually begin with the familiar and move to the unfamiliar. For example, in helping a woman who is a new diabetic to understand the principles of asepsis in the injection technique, the health teacher might draw on the woman's experience of infant feeding as a reference point.

Motivation for learning

Motivation is a crucial factor influencing learning. Lefrancois (1982) asks four questions which are related to motivation and learning:

- What initiates action?
- What directs behaviour?
- Why is behaviour learned?
- Why does behaviour stop? (p. 301)

There are a number of possible explanations for what motivates human behaviour. The first is instinct. However, instinct cannot fully account for complex human behaviours. Lefrancois (1982) writes that the notion of instincts may be more appropriate to the behaviour of animals than humans, and states:

> Perhaps a mother, left to her own devices, would instinctively know how to deliver and care for her child. Perhaps not. In any event, experience, culture, and evolution have so modified our behaviour that the question of the existence of human instinct has become largely irrelevant. (p. 304)

Other theories have been devised to explain learning behaviour in terms of needs and reactions to need. One, the need-drive theory, posits that when a physiological or psychological need occurs, it creates a state of arousal or energy which works to satisfy the need (Bernstein et al 2003). Frequently a motive is described in exactly those terms – as a force within that spurs the person to achieve in some direction.

Maslow (1943, 1970), in work that has become classic in this area, proposed a needs satisfaction theory according to which human beings strive to meet first their basic physiological needs and safety needs before concerning themselves with higher level needs (love, belongingness, self-esteem) culminating in the highest level need, self-actualization. The higher level needs are achieved through a personal, therefore idiosyncratic, desire to develop and grow. Maslow's theory is addressed more fully in Chapter 6 of this book.

Later, Weiner (1980) proposed a cognitive theory of motivation. In this theory people are considered as active participants in creating their own motivation through desire to learn or in anticipation of learning. The Gestalt cognitive theorists discussed earlier presented motivation as a tension or force created by the difference between what the individual desires and achieves. McClelland and his colleagues (1953) had developed an achievement motivation theory which is similar. Tensions set up within the individual force him to seek to achieve to the degree which will ease the tension. McClelland's work was further developed by Atkinson (1974) who recognized that motivation was also affected by a separate tendency to avoid failure. The need for achievement can motivate individuals to master learning tasks (Bernstein et al 2003).

All these theories assume that some degree of need exists, and that the need will excite a response that initiates behaviour to meet the need. Arousal is such a response and, in its simplest definition, refers to the degree of alertness within an individual. Visual and auditory senses are primary sources of arousal, and these can be enhanced by properties such as novelty and meaningfulness (Berlyne 1960). Optimal arousal (or attention to the learning task) is conducive to learning. In a person who is bored, little learning will occur.

Anxiety is related to the level of arousal, and at a high level it may be detrimental to learning. The young woman who has a stoma created in surgery for cancer of the bowel may be so worried about the recurrence of cancer that her learning to care for her stoma may be inhibited. The single mother living in deprived circumstances without social support may be too anxious to attend to information about why smoking is detrimental to her own and her child's health.

The mechanism of arousal can be controlled to a certain degree by manipulating those variables which are external to the individual. For instance, if

ACTIVITY 3.2

■ What subject that you have studied recently have you liked learning about most? Explore your motivation for this. Why did you like it and want to learn about it?

■ Think of a subject you have studied that you liked less. Since you didn't especially like it, what motivated you to want to learn about it?

■ Now see if you can categorize your sources of motivation. Which were 'intrinsic'? That is, which came from your own desire to learn or your interest in the subject itself? On the other hand, which were extrinsic? That is, which came from the expectation of external rewards, such as praise or a grade?

■ Which sources of motivation do you think were most effective in encouraging your learning?

vision is an arousal source, the use of audiovisual aids will stimulate the learners, though learning may also be enhanced by a lively voice and presentation style. One rule of thumb seems to be variety (Lefrancois 1982) to evoke optimal levels of arousal for learning.

Two kinds of motivation are distinguished by psychologists:

■ intrinsic motivation, which does not depend on any observable rewards or reinforcement, and

■ extrinsic motivation, which depends on reinforcement from the outside (Adams & Bromley 1998).

Motivation which is solely extrinsic persists only for a short period after reinforcement stops. The need to encourage the development of intrinsic motivation in health teaching is clear. The distinction between the two types of motivation helps to explain the low rate of compliance with prescribed regimes. In hospital, when reinforcement is provided by health professionals, the patient may simply comply without creating his own motivation by considering fully his health problem and its effects. With the withdrawal of reinforcement out of the hospital, the desired behaviour is likely to stop unless the patient has internalized the motivation to continue and therefore needs no external rewards.

The relationship of memory to learning

Early theories of learning were concerned with how change in knowledge and behaviour occurred. Theories about memory, on the other hand, deal with how knowledge is retained. In practice, memory and learning are very much interrelated. Any task of learning or memory depends upon the individual's ability to perceive and transform knowledge from the environment (sometimes 'encoding'), attend to information presented and retrieve information already stored in the memory. The individual's ability to retain knowledge influences the extent of comprehension and reasoning.

Memory is needed for individuals to maintain changed behaviour. In a person's memory are stored attitudes, skills and thinking strategies, all essential to learning.

In order to think, reason, learn, remember or recognize things as being meaningful or familiar, it is necessary to be able to store large quantities of information. Storage of information is one function of memory, but storage alone is not enough. Any store needs to be organized so that items held may be located and retrieved. Finding a book in a library or a drug in a medicine cupboard depends on the existence of a reliable retrieval system. In the library, this function is served by a catalogue; in the medicine cupboard it is served by an orderly system of organization that is understood by the persons who use it. Similarly, human memory functions by having a system whereby information stored may be classified or categorized and subsequently retrieved. Such a system may be dependent on the existence of different types of memory or levels of processing. Cognitive psychologists (e.g. Broadbent 1958, 1966) have identified a model of memory which contains two major elements, short-term memory (STM) and long-term memory (LTM) (Bernstein et al 2003).

- *The STM* holds a limited amount of material for a short time, and it also represents the working space in which problem solving is carried out. It does not commit knowledge for later retrieval. An example would be reading a number in a telephone directory and remembering it just long enough to dial the number. Often, if the number is engaged, the person has to look it up again, because it has already escaped from the STM. In class, students may be taking notes and making sense of them as they write them down, linking them with information they already know. But shortly after the class they may not be able to recall much of the material they have just recorded.

- *The LTM* is more stable and not as easily disturbed. That is to say, the memory is retained on a long-term basis. However, long-term memory is said to be constructive rather than simply reproductive, which means that the person's account of previous experience may be coloured or distorted. This is one explanation for the unreliability that may occur with eyewitnesses to crimes. One of the problems that has challenged psychologists and has yet to be resolved is how the information in the LTM is organized and how associative links are made between bits of information.

Information may be passed between short- and long-term memory, depending on its salience to the individual. The exact interrelationship of parts of the memory system is not known, but human memory is a multi-process operation and, whatever the storage system, memory seems to depend on how information is processed for storage (Kintsch 1977). People process information for storage according to their prior knowledge. One teenage boy hearing about the dangers of smoking might be thinking of his grandfather who smoked heavily and recently died of lung cancer, while another hearing the same information might be thinking of a much-admired snooker player who is always seen smoking between his turns at the table. The information stored in the LTMs of these two young men might be quite different, because they perceive the information according to different sets of prior experience.

Memory thus depends on the individual's being able to store and retrieve information and is enhanced according to the individual's ability to categorize and organize material in a meaningful way. Processes by which memory may be enhanced are by combining items, by forming associations with items, or by rehearsing (repeating them over and over). The amount and timing of rehearsals can be all-important in memory, as can knowledge of which items to rehearse. The practical applications of such features of memory are explored in Chapter 5 in relation to the presentation of factual information in health teaching.

People have their own individual approaches to processing information for remembering, and may remember best if allowed to use their own systems (Mandler & Pearlstone 1966). In general, however, events are best remembered if they are meaningful, organized, striking in a visual sense or overlearned. Various theories have been posited to account for forgetfulness, and these include the fading of memories not frequently recalled, the suppression of memories unpleasant to the individual, and a poorly organized retrieval system (Lefrancois 1982). A further theory that has been suggested is interference, which suggests that forgetting can occur in one of two ways: retroactively, that is, forgetting because something learned since has inhibited the memory; or proactively, that is, forgetting because previous learning has inhibited the memory (Entwistle 1988). In other words, sometimes prior learning adversely affects the ability to remember, other times it is subsequent learning which causes forgetting.

Learning styles

Much research has been done by educational researchers into styles of learning, and various theories have been postulated to account for individual differences in approach and outcome. These have particular relevance for health teaching because of the need to tailor such teaching to the individual needs and circumstances of the intended learner. Two such theories arising from seminal pieces of research in educational psychology are of particular interest.

Deep-level and surface-level processing

Marton and Säljö (1976) identified these two styles of learning based on studies carried out with university students. Deep-level processing occurred when students approached a learning task with the intention of understanding the meaning it contained, questioned any arguments within the material, and tried to relate the information to previous knowledge and experience. Surface-level processing took place when students' intention was to memorize the factual elements within the material, with a view to being able to reproduce the information they thought they would be questioned about afterwards. In brief, deep-level processing involves seeking understanding, while surface-level processing involves learning by rote (Rehm 1995).

Several points are worth noting in relation to these styles of learning. First, the labels are best applied to learning events rather than to individuals. That is, it is more useful to say that a learner used a deep- or surface-level approach in a given situation than to describe the learner as a deep- or surface-level processor (Biggs 1999; Shale & Trigwell 2003).

Second, there is a clear link between the context of learning and the approach adopted for learning. In part, the context is set by the nature of the learning task. In addition, however, the teacher's expectations play a significant role. For example, in a course assessed by a single end-of-year written examination in which students will be expected to reproduce factual material, students will learn to adopt a surface-level approach, because that is what they will be rewarded for. If, on the other hand, a course requires students to produce course work which demonstrates logical argument and original thinking, those students are more likely to adopt a deep-level approach.

A third point is that although for most purposes a deep-level approach achieves better learning, there are times when surface-level processing is useful. A simple example is the multiplication of numbers. It is important to understand the meaning of multiplication as an arithmetic process, or one cannot know when it is appropriate to multiply, but life is certainly easier if one has memorized the multiplication tables.

Serialist and holist strategies

These strategies were identified by Pask (1976) and colleagues, again in studies with university students. They discovered that in some cases, students tackled a learning task by adopting a step-by-step strategy, taking a linear route to the completion of the task. In other cases, students took a more global approach, first gaining an overall view of the total picture and then filling in the detail. Both strategies, if applied effectively, could lead to successful completion of learning, but further study identified 'pathologies of learning'. The pathology of the serialist strategy occurred when the learner was not able to put the steps together to achieve a successful learning result, a full and complete understanding of the learning required. The pathology of the holist strategy occurred when the learner jumped to conclusions or failed to establish the validity of the pieces of the learning puzzle, and so ended up with a flawed understanding.

As with the deep and surface approaches, it is better to label the approach used than to label the learner. Learners may have a preferred style, but they may be able to adopt either style, and this is probably the ideal. Pask refers to this ability as a 'versatile' style, meaning that the person can adopt either a serialist or holist approach depending on the requirements of the learning task.

In more recent work, Entwistle has developed these theories further. His work indicates that learners use their learning skills strategically, that is, they take whatever learning styles they possess and adapt them to the needs of the learning situation. Thus the context of the learning situation will affect the

ACTIVITY 3.3

■ Think of a new area of subject matter you have had to tackle in your studies. What sort of approach did you take to it? Did you set out to understand the material, or did you try to memorize the necessary facts and figures? See if you can identify the reasons for selecting the approach you used. Were they related to the nature of the subject matter, or did they represent a habitual way of working, for you? Whichever approach you used – deep-level or surface-level – can you think of an example of material you approached using the other type of processing?

■ Repeat the same exercise, but this time consider whether you tried to learn the material by taking a serialist or holist approach.

■ For the two pairs of learning styles – surface-level versus deep-level processing and serialist versus holist strategy – suggest examples of health topics you might teach to a patient or client and decide which member of each pair would represent an appropriate learning approach.

style the learner employs, and can therefore influence whether the learning is effective or not (Entwistle 1998, 2000).

While the studies mentioned above were largely carried out with university students, the insights they offer can be helpful when transferred to other types of learning contexts, such as learning for health.

The adult as learner

Recent educational research has suggested that adults learn differently from children, for a number of reasons which encompass aspects of the physical as well as the psychological state.

Physical effects of ageing

Although cognitive functioning does not necessarily decline with age, there are ageing effects which may in turn affect learning. Deterioration of vision becomes noticeable after the age of 40. The normal eye at the age of 20 admits twice the amount of light as does the pupil in a 50-year-old. Other vision deficits include decreased recovery from glare effects, slower accommodation to darkness and a gradual decrease in colour sensitivity. These changes may be critical, as much of what an individual learns is by sight. Hearing is affected by age, with a loss of auditory acuity for high-pitched sounds. The other senses of taste, touch and smell may decrease only gradually.

With age, psychomotor skill learning slows due to changes in the neuromuscular system. Reaction times increase and teachers find that older learners take longer to follow directions or to respond to questions. Accuracy does not diminish if the older individual is left to work at his or her own pace.

Short-term memory is also affected by ageing. The process is more prone to

TABLE 3.2	Summary of physical effects of ageing and compensatory actions
Physical effects of ageing	**Compensatory actions**
Vision	
Pupillary size ↓	If using printed material, print must be readable
Colour sensitivity ↓	Increase non-glare lighting
Recovery from glare ↓	Use strong colours in audiovisual aids (green, red, black)
Hearing	
↓ for high-pitched sounds	Speak distinctly, not shrilly
	Control environmental distractions
Psychomotor	
Reaction time ↑	Allow self-paced activity
Memory	
Short-term ↓	Keep directions to a minimum, reinforce oral instructions with written material
	Develop learning materials in manageable amounts

disruption by intervening activity. Again, by allowing individuals to pace themselves, the results can equal the performance of younger learners. Table 3.2 summarizes the physical changes occurring with ageing and suggests how to compensate for them in health teaching situations. It is important to remember that these are generalizations, and cannot be expected to apply equally and exactly in all cases.

Age and psychological manifestations

Jenny Rogers (2001) has noted a number of reactions which may be seen in the adult learner. The older learner may be anxious about appearing foolish if concepts or skills are not grasped quickly. Such risk-taking may not be seen as worthwhile since the adult's status and self-esteem may be threatened.

The question of risk to status and self-esteem has particular relevance in health teaching, since teaching so often takes place in situations such as a hospital, a surgery or clinic, in which people feel at a disadvantage, or in circumstances such as illness or uncertainty, which reduce confidence. Additionally, the person's usual claims to status based on occupation and socioeconomic position may be temporarily threatened, suspended, or at least not immediately obvious. Such considerations may all lead to lack of self-confidence in the learner, and thus present barriers to learning.

Another reaction contributing adversely to the learning process may be the individual's view of ageing. The person may believe that 'you can't teach an old dog new tricks'. In addition, memories of past learning experiences may colour the learner's motivation to participate. If learning has presented problems in the past there may be expectation of a further negative experience.

A final consideration in adult learning is social background. Social distance between teacher and learner may be more important in adults than in children. Additionally, adults will have formed attitudes as to how much control they have over their own destiny, and over illness in particular, to aspects of health and disease, and to learning itself. These attitudes will influence people's expectations of success in learning, and their willingness and ability to learn.

In recent years, increasing attention has been given to the notion of 'andragogy'. This term is used by Knowles (1984, 1990) to refer to the learning experience of adults, which he says should be differentiated from that of children. He suggests that the traditional approach to education, or pedagogy, has been geared to children's learning, and that its underlying assumptions are not relevant to adults. (More recently he has questioned whether they are really appropriate for children either.) He believes that traditional pedagogy assumes:

- that the learner is necessarily dependent, and the teacher must control all decisions about learning
- that learning has to do with receiving transmitted knowledge, so learners' experiences are irrelevant
- that readiness to learn is chronologically determined, and learners should progress from learning what is appropriate at one level to that which is appropriate at the next
- that learning should be subject- or content-centred; and

■ that the learner's motivation comes from external sources, such as parents and teachers.

On the other hand, Knowles suggests a contrasting set of assumptions that should be made about adults and their learning:

■ that learners are capable of self-direction and can and should take responsibility for their own learning
■ that learners have a vast store of experience, and that it is relevant to the learning context
■ that readiness to learn is related to the learner's perception of a need to learn
■ that learning should be life-centred and based around problem-solving experiences; and
■ that learners' motivation is strongly internal and based on a need for self-esteem and self-confidence.

Knowles' contribution to learning theory has much to offer the health teacher, since health teaching is so directly related to people's own experiences and must be put into operation by them in their own lives. In addition, the learning that is intended depends heavily on the learner's internal motivation, and therefore it must relate to the person's felt needs.

Readiness to learn

A complex network of factors within and around each individual influences that person's readiness to learn at any given time. Some of these factors are fairly obvious, such as age, intellectual capacity, educational level, and previous experience. The person's physical condition will also have an effect. A person who is hungry, thirsty, exhausted, or in pain is unlikely to be a receptive learner. Emotional factors are also important. Being anxious, worried, angry, or upset can act as a barrier to learning.

People may have preconceived ideas that influence their ability to understand and accept new knowledge about a topic. They may not take kindly to having long-cherished beliefs challenged. Sometimes such ideas or beliefs have been picked up without the person's being aware of having learned anything. This is an important point for the health teacher to be aware of, not only with respect to previously learned ideas, but also with respect to what is being learned in the current context. All learning is not deliberate; some is unintentional and virtually unconscious. Thus the health teacher may be bringing about learning without realizing it, and this learning may or may not be what the health teacher is intending to teach.

Vanetzian (1997 p. 593) offers a useful basic definition of learning readiness that suits the health teaching context:

[Learning readiness is] evidence of motivation and ability to learn at a particular time; a dynamic state that influences the outcomes of patient teaching.

She refers to achievement motivation, described by Atkinson (1983), as being an important consideration. It is suggested that individuals are more motivated to try to succeed at learning when the learning task is neither to easy nor too difficult, and when it is possible to predict the level of difficulty. She also mentions factors such as 'level of anxiety, fatigue, depression, hope and perception of quality of life' (Vanetzian 1997 p. 593). Thus people are more ready to learn when they are not overly anxious, tired or depressed, and when they perceive that their quality of life may be improved for the better through the learning, and when they believe they will be able to succeed in achieving the learning.

A person's stage of development may have a significant influence on his or her ability or readiness to learn. Perry (1970, 1988) has described a scheme of intellectual and ethical development which is useful for the health teacher to consider. He identifies nine positions on a dimension, starting from Position 1, in which the individual believes in absolutes. There is clear right and wrong, good and bad, and these are related to 'us and them' – what 'we' know or believe is right and good. For the learner, the implication of this is that correct learning can be gained from those of 'us' in authority: parents, teachers, clergymen and the like.

As time goes on and the individual discovers that there are things that those in authority don't always agree about or know, the person moves by stages toward the pivotal position, Position 5. At this position the individual no longer believes that anything is absolute or certain, but that all knowledge and values are relative and context-dependent (Shale & Trigwell 2003). This position cannot be sustained, however, and again by stages the individual discovers that choices and decisions have to be made, even in the absence of certainty. Some decisions are better than others, and all decisions have consequences, and at the final position, Position 9, the individual has learned to make commitments, accept the consequences of those commitments, and accept the fact that others have different opinions and make different choices. Perry describes this position as 'contextual relativistic reasoning' (Perry 1970).

Perry's scheme has obvious implications for learning about health. For example, a person at one of the early developmental positions may accept information from someone in authority virtually unquestioningly, whereas a person at a later developmental position may be more questioning. It could be said that the ideal would be to facilitate the individual's development towards Position 9 with respect to his learning and understanding about health.

Fostering learning

Learning can be a challenging, satisfying and sometimes painful experience. The individual who becomes personally involved in his or her health, and is motivated to act responsibly and creatively, illustrates the ultimate aim of health teachers.

It has been shown that the learning and teaching process is an interactive one, a mutual process. To achieve this sense of mutuality, a commitment is required from both participants and should include personal involvement with ideas, the programme and each other, as well as others. The ultimate goal of learning about health is for the learner not only to gain knowledge but also to develop as a person. To foster such learning, the learner needs the teacher to be sincere and genuine, a person with vitality, convictions and feelings. Being cared for, valued, and accepted as a unique individual all contribute to the success of the learning experience.

ACTIVITY 3.4

- In relation to Perry's scheme, can you identify your own position of intellectual/ethical development? In doing this, it might be helpful to consider whether you can place yourself at a single position for all purposes, or whether you might be at a different position with respect to different specific aspects of your development.

- Consider the issue of abortion. How might it be viewed by a person who is at Position 1 in Perry's scheme of development? How would this differ from the way it might be viewed by a person at Position 5? Can you suggest how the person might move onwards towards Position 9? What kinds of experiences and thinking might accompany that development?

- Finally, here is a thorny problem: Perry's scheme seems to imply that the development from Position 1 to Position 9 is a 'good thing', that it represents the positive development of maturity. If you accept that viewpoint, have you taken a stand that is characteristic of Position 1 thinking? Or is it possible to arrive at Position 9, yet hold clear ideas about good and bad, right and wrong? (It is only fair to note that Perry did not suggest his scheme as a prescription, as what should happen; it represented a description of a phenomenon he identified through a series of interviews with individuals over a four-year period, that is, an organized account of what did happen.)

The above discussion has implications for the nurse as health teacher. The health teacher needs to use encounters to listen and to communicate, not to self-articulate. Nurses who seek to teach for health must be reliable, consistent and have a strong self-concept which can admit to error. They are committed to health and to teaching as a way to enhance life. They are flexible and able to accept new ideas, changes and challenges from the learners and from contemporaries. These are demanding requirements, but no more so than other qualities expected of health professionals.

Effective health teaching occurs in an environment that is supportive, non-judgemental and unhurried, and in which the learners are encouraged and facilitated to develop in ways that are most meaningful to them. Learners who have experienced the best of what health teaching can do leave the learning situation and:

- value their own worth, their feelings and reactions
- have faith in their own ability to achieve
- gain insight into their own motivation and behaviour
- feel responsible for themselves and others
- have experienced freedom through self-direction in learning, and
- gain satisfaction from the learning.

The remaining chapters address the ways in which the nurse as health teacher can seek to facilitate such learning.

REFERENCES

Adams B , Bromley B 1998 Psychology for Health Care – Key Terms and Concepts. Macmillan, Basingstoke.

Atkinson JW 1983 Personality, motivation and action: selected papers. Preager, New York.

Ausubel DP 1968 Educational psychology: a cognitive view. Holt Rinehart and Winston, New York.

Ausubel DP, Novak JS, Hanesian H 1978 Educational psychology: a cognitive view, 2nd edn. Holt Rinehart and Winston, New York.

Berlyne DE 1960 Conflict, arousal and curiosity. McGraw-Hill, New York.

Bernstein D, Clarke-Stewart A, Penner LA, Roy EJ 2003 Psychology. Houghton Mifflin, Boston.

Biggs J 1999 Teaching for quality learning at university. Open University Press, Buckingham.

Bloom B S (ed) 1956 Taxonomy of educational objectives, handbook I: cognitive domain. David McKay, New York.

Broadbent DE 1958 Perception and communication. Pergamon, London.

Broadbent DE 1966 The well ordered mind. American Educational Research Journal 3: 281-295.

Bruner JS 1960 The process of education. Harvard University Press, Cambridge Massachusetts.

Bruner JS 1964 The course of cognitive growth. American Psychologist 19: 1-15.

Entwistle N 1988 Styles of learning and teaching. David Fulton, London.

Entwistle NJ 1998 Improving teaching through research on student learning. In: Forest JJF (ed) University Teaching: Internatiional Perspectives. Garland publishing, New York.

Entwistle NJ 2000 Approaches to studying and levels of understanding: The influences of teaching and assessment. In: Smart J C (ed) Higher education: Handbook of theory and research, Vol 15 (pages 156-218). Agathon Press, New York.

Funderstanding 1998-2001 http://www.funderstanding.com/constructivism.cfm 10.8.03 Accessed March 19, 2003.

Gagné RM 1974 Essentials of learning for instruction. Dryden Press, Hinsdale, Illinois.

Hartley J 1998 Learning and studying. Routledge, London.

Kintsch W 1977 Memory and cognition. John Wiley, New York.

Knowles M 1984 Andragogy in action. Jossey Bass, San Francisco.

Knowles MS 1990 The adult learner – a neglected species, 4th edn. Gulf Publishing, Houston.

Koffka K 1935 Principles of gestalt psychology. International Library of Psychology, Philosophy and Scientific Method, London.

Köhler W 1929 Gestalt psychology. Liveright, New York.

Krathwohl DK, Bloom BS, Masia BB 1964 Taxonomy of educational objectives, handbook II: affective domain. David McKay, New York.

Lefrancois GR 1982 Psychology for teaching, 4th edn. Wadsworth, Belmont California.

McClelland DC, Atkinson W, Clark RA, Lowell EL 1953 The achievement motive. Appleton-Century-Crofts, New York.

Mandler G, Pearlstone Z 1966 Free and constrained concept learning and subsequent recall. Journal of Verbal Learning and Verbal Behaviour 5: 126-131.

Marton F, Säljö R 1976 On qualitative differences in learning 1: outcome and process. British Journal of Educational Psychology 46: 4-11.

Maslovaty N & Kuzi E 2002 Promoting motivational goals through alternative of traditional assessment. Studies in Educational Evaluation 28: 199-222.

Maslow AH 1943 A theory of human motivation. Psychological Review 501:370-396.

Maslow AH 1970 Motivation and personality, 2nd edn. Harper & Row, New York.

Nisbet J, Shucksmith J 1986 Learning strategies. Routledge & Kegan Paul, London.

Pask G 1976 Styles and strategies of learning. British Journal of Educational Psychology 46: 128-148.

Perry WG 1970 Forms of intellectual and ethical development in the college years: a scheme. Holt Rinehart and Winston, New York.

Perry WG 1988 Different worlds in the same classroom. In: Ramsden P (ed) Improving learning: new perspectives. Kogan Page, London.

Rehm J 1995 Deep/Surface Approaches to Learning: An Introduction. National Teaching and Learning Forum 5(1): . http://www.ntlf.com/html/pi/9512/article1.htm Accessed August 15, 2003.

Rogers C 1969 Freedom to learn. Merrill, New York.

Rogers C, Freiberg H G 1994 Freedom to learn, 3rd edn. Merrill, Columbus Ohio.

Rogers J 2001 Adults learning, 4th edn. Open University Press, Milton Keynes.

Romiszowski AJ 1988 Designing instructional systems: decision making in course planning and curriculum design. Kogan Page, London.

Shale S, Trigwell K 2003 Paper 2: Student approaches to learning. Institute for the Advancement of University Learning, Oxford http://www.learning.ox.ac.uk/iaul/IAUL+1+2+3.asp Accessed September 5, 2003.

Skinner BF 1953 Science and human behaviour. Macmillan, New York.

Smith MK (1999) The social/situational orientation to learning. In: infed, the encyclopedia of informal education http://www.infed.org/biblio/learning-social.htm Accessed September 7, 2003.

Vanetzian E 1997 Learning readiness for patient teaching in stroke rehabilitation. Journal of Advanced Nursing 26(3): 589-594.

Weiner B 1980 Human motivation. Holt, Rinehart and Winston, New York.

4 Therapeutic and persuasive communication

The process of communication is central to the teaching–learning process. The word communication connotes sharing. To communicate means to represent a message and send it to another person through a medium such as sight, smell, taste, touch or hearing. The process is dynamic and it occurs constantly, whether or not we are aware of it.

Communication may be oral or written, verbal, nonverbal or extraverbal (paraverbal). All interaction involves communication. Talking with a friend, waving at a neighbour in the street, explaining an ailment to the doctor, sharing grief at the death of a favourite pet, sending an E-mail message to friends to arrange a party, debating a problem with fellow students in a tutorial group, widening one's eyes in surprise, nodding one's head in agreement, indicating to turn left in a car – all involve communication. What was said? How was it said? What was meant? What was implied with words? What was implied without words? How was the message received by the person to whom it was directed? Was the meaning inferred by the receiver the same as the meaning intended by the sender? Such questions illustrate that communication is not mere 'talk', but a complex process which can lead to misunderstanding as well as understanding.

Communication is thus a two-way process, involving the passing of messages back and forth between a sender and a receiver. Figure 4.1 illustrates a simple model of communication.

Communication plays an important role in nursing. Nurses have to be skilled communicators in order to identify patients' or clients' needs, assist in the expression of needs, aid the understanding of preventive activity, treatment or care, and facilitate the acquisition of self-care skills. To be effective communicators, nurses have to be skilled receivers as well as senders of messages.

FIGURE 4.1   *A communication model*

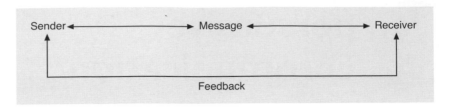

In health education, communication is a planned process which is effective when the client attains certain goals. Health teaching is integral to the normal process of therapeutic communication between nurse and patient.

THERAPEUTIC COMMUNICATION

Therapeutic communication in nursing has been described by Gazda et al (1975, 1999) as a three-phase cycle of helping, involving facilitation, transition and action. The essential features of the facilitation phase are talking and listening in a manner that is empathetic, warm, non-directive and non-judgemental. It is important to respect the individual and to accept his interpretation of events. Such an approach reduces feelings of threat and the client is able to speak freely, release emotions and explore the problem. The basis of the therapeutic relationship is thus laid.

The transition phase requires more intervention. When the patient has reached saturation point and cannot take self-exploration and understanding any further without help, the nurse can ask specific relevant questions. At this point the nurse needs to demonstrate interest and genuineness, and may use self-disclosure if such a tactic is appropriate. However, the nurse should be wary of expressions such as 'I know just how you feel', as they may communicate a message that the patient is not being seen as an individual or that his or her feelings are being discounted or trivialized. In the transition phase the patient's problem is defined.

In the action phase, problem solving begins. The nurse helps the patient to plan strategies. Confrontation about discrepancies in what the patient says or does may be needed. The patient who says, 'I know I'm overweight and I'm going to stick to a diet', but who continues to eat sweets regularly, may be confronted providing he or she has explored and understands his or her motivations for action.

In all helping relationships, termination must occur. Throughout the process of helping, both participants are learning about one another, the situation and the problem. A relationship is formed and must be ended when the patient no longer requires the help of the nurse, or when that help is in danger of leading to inappropriate dependence (see Figure 4.2).

It is all too easy to represent therapeutic communication as a straightforward sequential process and an easily acquired skill. In fact, for most nurses, it means acquiring new skills and trying to break old habits. In the first trial of a

FIGURE 4.2	*The phases of therapeutic communication*

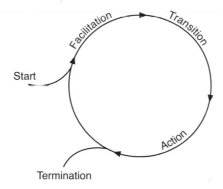

new skill such as bathing a patient or changing a dressing, the nurse may find the movements awkward. He or she may have to stop and think about principles and procedures and the whole process moves rather slowly. Eventually, with practice, the nurse becomes adept. Competence in the process of communicating therapeutically is attained in the same way. Awkwardness and artificiality accompany the first few efforts. With practice and regular review, the skill becomes smoother, easier and more effective.

THE COMMUNICATION PROCESS

Analysis of what happens in given communications can provide clues to understanding the process of communication. Consider, for instance, the following excerpt from a conversation between a staff nurse (female) from a general surgical ward and a preoperative patient:

> **Nurse** (on entering hospital room at 6:30 p.m.): 'Good evening, Mr Keighley. I've come to talk with you about your operation.'
>
> **Mr Keighley** (looking worried): 'Is there anything wrong? I mean, is everything still on for tomorrow?'
>
> **Nurse** (brightly): 'Oh, yes, the operation is still scheduled for tomorrow. I've come to explain some of the procedures that will occur before the operation and to answer any questions you might have.'
>
> **Mr Keighley**: 'Oh, that's all right, then.'

Elements of communication

In the above exchange there are six identifiable elements:

1 *The motivating reason for the exchange*: The nurse approached Mr Keighley for preoperative preparation and her reason was the need to communicate about what he should expect before and after surgery.

2   *The sender, or the person initiating the conversation, in this case the nurse*: How the nurse converses will be affected by her level of skill in communicating, her knowledge of the patient, her attitude towards the situation, her level of knowledge about the surgical procedure, and her sociocultural background, which includes her professional preparation.

3   *The message, which is the actual expression relayed to the other person*: How it is conveyed is important. Does it make sense or is it a jumble of words? Has there been a decision about the content? Will reference be made to professional jargon, such as 'preoperative procedures' or 'reducing surgical risks'? The content of the message must be closely considered to ensure that the patient is not left in confusion.

4   *The channel, which refers to the way the message is sent*: In the example, the nurse presented herself to Mr Keighley and spoke to him, thereby stimulating the senses of sight and hearing.

5   *The receiver, that is, the person to whom the message is directed*: The message has to be received and understood. If Mr Keighley had not seen or heard the nurse entering the room, or had not recognized that she was addressing him, he would not have acted as receiver and would not have understood the message. Similarly, if he had been distracted or uninterested, he might not have 'received' the message the nurse was intending to send. The receiver's communication skills, knowledge level, attitudes and sociocultural background all influence how he participates, how he comprehends what is being said to him.

6   *Feedback, the final stage*: In this stage, Mr Keighley responded to the nurse to let her know he understood that she was speaking to him on a particular topic, his scheduled surgery, and what the purpose of the conversation was to be.

Figure 4.3 depicts a model of the communication process. The arrows in the figure depict a full circle to indicate that the receiver hears the message. The

---

FIGURE 4.3   *Model illustrating the process of communication*

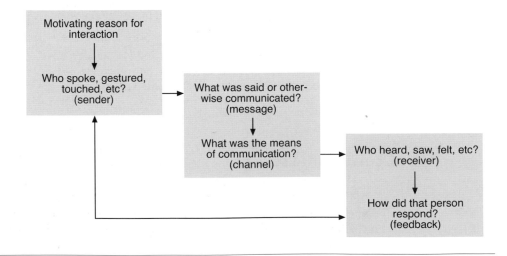

feedback to the sender might be 'I understand', or 'I don't understand', or 'Can you repeat that?' In this way the process is completed. It may then recommence. If the receiver responds (gives feedback) and adds something that sends a message that calls for a response, then the original sender becomes a receiver. In the example above, if in the course of the interaction about his surgery, Mr Keighley tells the nurse that he has an allergy to adhesive tape, at that point he is the sender and the nurse is the receiver. The process is dynamic and messages can be sent in both directions, alternately or at the same time. Figure 4.3 illustrates such a situation.

The dynamic of communication

While the spoken word is sometimes considered to be the major means of communicating, there are many other means. To distinguish the different aspects of communication, the term 'verbal' refers to the words used, 'paraverbal' or 'extraverbal' describes *how* words are said, and 'nonverbal' indicates all other means that achieve communication, including body language. Paraverbal and nonverbal modes may be just as important as verbal communication.

As an example of paraverbal or extraverbal communication, consider a patient who says to a nurse, 'I can't do what you're asking. It's impossible.' This sentence will be interpreted differently depending on whether the patient says it calmly, or loudly, or sobbing, or aggressively. The way the voice is used – the volume, the tone, the tempo, the emphasis, non-word sound effects – helps to convey what the patient means. Fiction writers have to find ways to express the paraverbal aspect of their characters' speech, otherwise the conversations would be flat. Another example of the challenge presented by paraverbal communication occurs when a researcher tries to transcribe verbatim the content of an interview with a research subject. In such cases, to omit the paraverbal elements can mean missing the real meaning or important subtleties in a piece of communication.

Nonverbal communication may entail means as widely varied as the use of pictures and the throwing of tantrums. An everyday and ever-present form of nonverbal communication is body language. This refers to messages communicated by the way a person stands, makes gestures, touches others, dresses, or adopts a position in relation to others. The use of nonverbal communication may be conscious, such as letting someone know by your facial expression that you are angry with him, or unconscious, such as when a person is feeling sad but is unaware that other people have noticed.

Nonverbal communication can be a clear and forceful way to convey, complement or emphasize a message, and at times it can express more than the sender realises. It can be particularly useful in situations where words are inadequate.

It is important, however, to be alert to the possibility of misinterpretation. A person who appears to be frowning, for example, may be squinting because of nearsightedness. In addition, there are cultural variations for many types of body language (Burton & Dimbleby 1995), so it is important for the health professional to be cautious before jumping to conclusions about the meanings of such symbolic aspects of communication. As Hanson (1996) points out, non-verbal cues should be assessed along with the person's verbal communication, rather than these being treated as separate variables.

TECHNIQUES OF THERAPEUTIC COMMUNICATION

While a number of techniques are utilized in therapeutic communication and are referred to in this chapter, three techniques are more fully described here because they constitute essential aspects of communication. These are questioning, listening and the use of silence, and interviewing. These devices are not discrete, but it is useful to address them individually.

Questioning

Questioning is a skill that can help:

- gain information about the patient's or client's level of knowledge, attitudes, opinions and feelings
- focus on particular subject matter
- express an interest or indicate attention
- involve the other person
- encourage self-exploration
- hold attention
- validate facts and observations
- clarify meanings.

The type of question asked may influence its effects. An *open-ended* question allows someone to describe or to elaborate on a topic. The nurse might ask, 'What is your pain like?' A *closed* question asks for specific information and limits the type of answer that can be given. A patient who has come into an accident and emergency department after sustaining a leg injury might be asked, 'Does your leg hurt?' to which the answer can only be 'yes' or 'no', or possibly some slight variation such as 'A little bit' or 'Yes, it's really bad'. *Leading* questions do just what they describe: they lead the respondent to give an answer that might not have been given spontaneously. They tend to elicit 'correct' responses: 'You aren't having any pain at the moment, are you?' This type of question is usually not helpful in achieving real communication. A *probing* question seeks further information. An example of the use of probing questions might be: 'You say it doesn't hurt as much as it did before. When do you mean? ... What was the pain like then? ... How is it different now?'

Questioning may sometimes come across as prying or threatening on the part of the nurse, particularly if the topic is something the patient or client feels sensitive about, such as sexual behaviour, or the amount the patient smokes or drinks. It is therefore important to respect the patient's dignity when introducing such subjects and to handle them with tact.

Listening and the use of silence

To meet a patient or client's needs, it is important to listen and to take account of what he or she says. Effective listening is not simply a passive thing. It requires that the nurse pay attention and show that he or she is paying attention. This can be achieved through body language, facial expression, eye contact, spoken cues such as 'Mm-hmm' or 'I see', or simply being silent to allow the other person the chance to speak.

The skilful use of silence can enhance effective communication. Silences in conversation may be uncomfortable, but in therapeutic communication they serve a useful purpose as they can give the patient time to think, to remember, or to formulate a response. Sometimes silence is a natural pause in the flow of the talking; at other times, it creates a feeling of embarrassment. During silence, the nurse can observe the patient's nonverbal behaviour and maintain an attitude which invites the other person to go on talking. As a paraverbal technique, silence can communicate that the nurse has time for the patient. It can be difficult to judge when silence would be both comfortable and appropriate but it is important not to assume that every pause should be filled with talk.

Interviewing types and techniques

Effective interviewing requires the use of both questioning and listening skills. The interview in health teaching is a process in which understanding of a situation is gained through the collection of information from the individual who is then helped to make decisions about his health status and/or his health-related behaviour. Garrett (1972 p. 5) has noted:

> Warm human interest does sometimes vanish from interviewing, and when that happens it becomes a monotonous, mechanical sort of thing that is relatively valueless. But the cause of this kind of interviewing, when it occurs, is (...) ignorance that regards interviewing as a routine affair of asking set questions and recording answers.

Thus, the interview should be conducted within an atmosphere of support in which rapport between the nurse and patient or client facilitates self-exploration. The amount of self-exploration depends on the purpose of the interview. Three types of interviewing illustrate different purposes.

The structured interview

This is conducted to obtain specific information. The nurse controls the pace of the interview, often asking closed questions. This type of interview has a particular place in crisis situations and with people who are acutely ill, where a leisurely talk will not provide essential details about the person sufficiently quickly.

The semi-structured interview

This can be used not only to gain information but also to explore feelings or to promote patient participation. For instance, when caring for antenatal clients, the midwife will want to know how the pregnancy is progressing and will collect information on, for example, weight, diet, physical changes. However, the feelings of the expectant woman will also be important. Does she want this baby? Is she having any fears about the labour and delivery period? What are the views of the baby's father? Such concerns can be probed by encouraging the client to talk. In such an interview only some of the questions, or the basic framework of the interview, are decided in advance. Open questions are used strategically to provide opportunities for the client to influence the direction of the interview so that it addresses her own concerns and needs.

The unstructured interview

In this type of interview, the direction of the agenda is largely in the control of the client or patient. Such an approach can be particularly valuable in exploring attitudes, feelings and values. The health visitor who would like to help secondary school students explore how they see health in relation to themselves can use an unstructured format. He or she will not want to force certain values and attitudes on the students, but will want them to question themselves about their own level of health, so questions are not determined in advance, but are allowed to arise. The unstructured interview can be challenging, because the nurse may find it difficult to give over control to the patient or client. In addition, there is a fine balance to be achieved in allowing the interview to progress along lines that serve the concerns of the client without letting it lose its purpose.

Many interviews contain elements of all three of these types. For example, an interview may begin with a structured set of questions, then move to a less structured format as wider issues are explored. In another case, an interview may begin in an unstructured, conversational style, and before it closes, it may become more structured as the nurse asks specific questions to be sure all the necessary information has been gained.

As a communication tool, the interview should reflect the pattern of facilitation, transition and action described for therapeutic communication.

- *Set the stage.* The interview begins by attending to the setting factors (furniture, lighting, privacy), by putting the patient or client at ease and offering openings to begin the exchange. The nurse facilitates the process by being empathetic, warm, encouraging and respectful.

- *Build on the work started.* Questioning can help the patient explore the problem, decide what the problem is, and make decisions about acting on it. The nurse maintains an attitude of interest, listens actively to what the patient says, and remains non-judgemental.

- *Close the interview.* Nursing interviews frequently have time limits. Keeping this in mind is important, as an abrupt departure from the patient may be unsettling and can destroy the trust which has been built up. There should be time to review what has been discussed, to summarize the state of affairs, to note what progress has been made, and to focus on finishing. Asking the patient, 'Is there anything else you'd like to say today?' allows him the choice of terminating and tells him that the exchange can continue if that is needed and appropriate.

At the end of an interview its effectiveness and results should be evaluated. What helpful information emerged? What was the patient's behaviour? Was the problem situation identified? What decisions were made? How should this information influence the care plan, including the teaching plan?

Interviewing is a skill which, like many others, is not easy at the outset but improves with practice. Certain behaviours which are detrimental to effective communication are common when a person is new at interviewing, and the nurse needs to learn to avoid these. Other behaviours are conducive to effective interviewing, and it is important to reinforce and develop these. Thus, one purpose of the evaluation at the end of an interview is reflection on practice – in this case, on the nurse's own interview technique.

ACTIVITY 4.1

Select an everyday health topic, then find a volunteer among your family or friends to act as interviewee. Using a tape recorder, conduct an interview in which you explore your selected topic with your 'client'. When you have finished, play the tape back and listen to yourself and your interviewee. Make notes on the strengths and weaknesses of your interview technique. In doing this, consider the following questions, making notes of your answers:

■ Who did most of the talking? Did you talk too much?

■ What kinds of questions did you ask? Were they open or closed?

■ Was your interviewee free to give his or her own answers, or did you suggest certain answers by the way you phrased the questions?

■ Did you follow up on cues your interviewee offered that warranted further exploration, or did you miss cues?

■ Did you actually listen to what the interviewee said, or did you sometimes miss the point by failing to allow sufficient time, or by thinking ahead to the next question on your agenda?

You may think of additional points of evaluation as you listen to your tape. Remember not to concentrate only on the shortcomings of your interview technique: It is equally important to be aware of the positive features. Repeat this exercise with a different 'volunteer', focusing on the points you noted from the first interview, and then listen again and evaluate your progress.

PERSUASIVE COMMUNICATION

Sooner or later every nurse involved in health teaching will face the challenge of deciding whether or not it is right to persuade others to change their behaviour, and how to achieve persuasion if this seems necessary or desirable.

In today's society everyone has experience of persuasion, either as persuader or as recipient of a would-be persuasive message. Ideas abound as to what will persuade: choose arguments to fit the target audience; get the language and pronunciation right; use vivid descriptions and good anecdotes; vary the tone of voice and manipulate body language; exploit rhyme and rhythm, figures of speech, cliché and paradox; demonstrate authority; amuse; charm; appeal to reason or to the emotions – these are all familiar tricks in daily use in techniques of political persuasion and commercial advertising.

Visual impact is another important aspect of persuasion: consider the symbolism of the cross and the swastika, for example. Today, television and Internet sites are among the most obvious exploiters of visual impact, but ancillary media such as badges, beer mats, pens, key-rings, T-shirts, designer labels, and many others are used to sell a product or an image. The emotive

BOX 4.1	*Three main approaches to persuasion among health educators*

Education	■ EXPLORE attitudes and behaviour ■ REWARD change
Propaganda	■ MANIPULATE attitudes and behaviour
Community development	■ ASSIST discovery of attitudes and behaviour ■ ACCEPT the initiation or rejection of change

power of music is also exploited, as is its power to be retained and associated with particular images. Most people can recall certain advertising jingles, even if they have never bought the particular products. Other techniques widely believed to be successful in persuasion include repetition, enthusiasm, intimidation and audience participation.

The link between beliefs, attitudes and behaviour

In health education, persuasive techniques are directed at bringing about changes in attitudes or behaviour. Broadly, there are three sets of assumptions made about how this may be done. These are reflected in three approaches to persuasion among health educators. Box 4.1 lists these approaches, all of which have two things in common. First, there is the assumption that beliefs, attitudes and behaviour are central to persuading people to change actions related to health. Second, it is implied that there is some link between belief, attitude and behaviour.

It is beyond the scope of this text to deal with the details of defining terms such as belief and attitude, but in considering persuasion it is useful for practical purposes to address the relationship between attitudes, beliefs and behaviour. This is neatly expressed by Blaxter (1990) in relation to her survey of health and lifestyle:

> at this point the question arises of beliefs, defined as those things which people know or think to be true. Correct beliefs are a necessary preliminary to taking effective action, but beliefs do not necessarily predict either attitudes or behaviour. The great majority of the population (...) believe that smoking is a cause of lung cancer. Holding this belief was only weakly associated with attitudes to smoking, however, and not at all with actually being a smoker or not. (...) In spite of these problematic issues, it is clear that some interaction of values, beliefs, and perceptions of costs and benefits, modified by both external situations and by personality factors, must influence behaviour. (pp. 148-149)

These factors have implications for the use of persuasion in health education. Researchers looking at persuasive communication have been challenged by the question of exactly how beliefs, attitudes and behaviour are linked. Traditional health education approaches have assumed that knowledge precedes attitudes and will both predict and precede behaviour. The Knowledge-Attitude-Practice

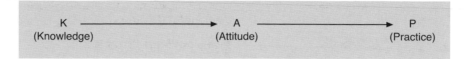

FIGURE 4.4   *The KAP model for health education*

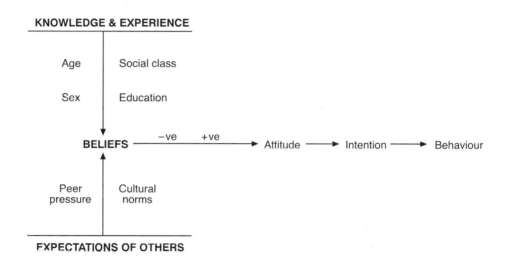

FIGURE 4.5   *The relationship of beliefs, attitudes, intentions and behaviour*

(KAP) model of health education is an example of this assumption. Figure 4.4 illustrates the simple KAP model. The model suggests that the right information will influence attitudes and thus change behaviour (practice). As is shown in the quotation above, this approach is naive and the relationship between knowledge, attitudes and behaviour is more complex. Some types of information change some people's attitudes some of the time, but the knowledge-attitude-behaviour link is neither consistent nor unidirectional. Changing attitudes does not seem to guarantee a change in behaviour. Additionally, it is known that changes in behaviour may bring about changes in attitude.

Fishbein and Ajzen (1981) have proposed that clusters of beliefs influence the formation of specific attitudes which in turn determine an individual's intention to act. Figure 4.5 illustrates this idea. Everyday experience, however, indicates that people do not always behave as they intend. The gap between intention and behaviour remains the major challenge to health educators. Somewhere in that gap there is an as yet unexplained interaction of strength of motivation versus the context in which health-related actions take place (Figure 4.6).

For a time, the idea of any attitude-behaviour link was seriously questioned by researchers. Some research studies appeared to demonstrate that attitudes were not reliable predictors of behaviour. The first and perhaps most famous of

FIGURE 4.6   *The intention–behaviour gap*

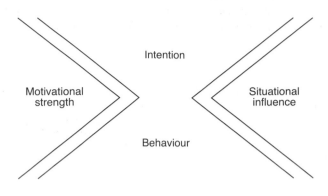

these was published by La Piere (1934). He recorded that when a Chinese couple accompanied by a Caucasian toured restaurants and hotels in the USA they were refused admission at only one of 251 establishments. This was despite the fact that 92% of the owners said in response to a postal survey that they would not admit Chinese. Thus, doubt was cast on the assumed link between attitude and behaviour. However, later reviews of the research (Ajzen & Fishbein 1977; Petty et al 1981) revealed that shortcomings in research design and methodology may account for the inconsistencies between attitude and behaviour that have been recorded. Firstly, attitudes are very difficult to measure and some researchers have opted for recording a verbal report of the attitude, which may or may not be the same as the attitude itself. Other aspects of some of the studies can also be questioned. For instance, in the La Piere case, it is possible that managers handled the written query about reservations but other staff members dealt with the face-to-face encounters. Clearly, if different people were sampled there would be no reason to expect an attitude-behaviour link. Petty et al (1981) conclude that it can be assumed that there is, after all, a link between attitude and behaviour. What cannot be assumed is that the link is either linear or simple. Nonetheless, for all practical purposes it can be accepted that attempting to form and change attitudes remains a worthwhile pursuit of those who wish to influence health-related behaviour.

Theories relevant to the formation of attitudes

Since persuasive communication still may be legitimately concerned with attitude change or attitude formation, it is necessary to examine the contribution of some major theories to ideas about how attitudes are formed and changed.

Behaviourist learning theories

Behaviourist learning theories (described in Chapter 3) would suggest that attitudes are changed as individuals respond to rewards and punishments. Thus, the principles of classical and operant conditioning may be applied to attitude formation and change. Learning to associate positive and negative attitudes with a given health behaviour is assumed to be what motivates the individual to adopt or reject the behaviour. For instance, in dental health education it is common to concentrate on the aesthetic aspects of good teeth, on the assumption that a person who believes good teeth are attractive will develop positive attitudes to dental care.

Functional theories

Functional theories emphasize the relationship of persuasive communication to the person's underlying personality and motivational needs. Katz (1960) has proposed that attitudes may serve four functions for the individual:

- *instructional function*: to satisfy physical, social, emotional and intellectual needs
- *ego defence function*: to protect the self-image, help the individual deal with conflicts
- *value expressive function*: to give expression to self-concept and self-identity
- *knowledge function*: to give meaning, by providing the individual with order and stability.

Other needs have been suggested, but all functionalists suggest that attitudes emerge to meet personal or social needs and that attitudes change when they are no longer functional. According to functional theory, then, for a communication to succeed in persuading, it must address the function of the attitude to be changed. For instance, take the example of a man who needs to feel superior towards women and holds a belief, based on that need, that women are inferior drivers. Factual information, even the best-researched evidence, will be unlikely to change his attitude to women drivers. In this case, persuasion will depend upon being able to help him identify and remove his need to feel superior.

Perceptual theories

Perceptual theories suggest that how the individual perceives a communication will affect whether or not he is persuaded by it. Underlying a person's perception are various factors that affect that perception.

Obviously, perception is affected by a range of physical factors such as acuity of sight or hearing. It will also be affected by psychological factors such as mood or state of anxiety. In the cognitive realm, the individual's level of intellectual ability, knowledge and understanding will affect how things in the environment are perceived. Other factors that may be influential include cultural background, upbringing, group and peer pressure.

Adams and Bromley make the point that 'We pay attention to things that have importance for us individually, depending on our needs and interests' (1998 p. 209). It could be further suggested that people take what they want out of a message and that they listen best to things they want to hear.

Consistency theories

Consistency theories propose that the individual will strive to keep harmony within his internal belief system, and that attitude change results from the need to make adjustments to restore or maintain harmony. That is, attitudes change when some fact, behaviour or event causes inconsistency or imbalance within the belief system. These theories came into prominence in the 1950s.

One theory that has applied the idea of balance to identifying what occurs in persuasion is Osgood et al's *congruity theory* (Osgood & Tannenbaum 1955; Osgood et al 1957). This theory suggests that if someone has a positive attitude towards a person and a negative attitude to a particular event or object, he is likely to draw those two attitudes together if he finds out that the person he admires feels positively towards the event or idea he dislikes. He will either develop a less favourable attitude to the person or a more favourable attitude to the event or idea. In other words, he will shift his attitudes to make them more congruent. The theory predicts that if attitude change is necessary to restore congruity, then both attitudes will change, the more extreme attitude changing least.

Congruity theory, then, suggests that having a high regard for a message communicator may influence the person to change his attitudes, provided his positive attitude to the communicator is stronger than his negative attitudes to the position advocated. If someone feels strongly about a particular issue and his views clash with the advocate of that position, it is possible that he will review his opinion of the individual concerned, if that is the less strongly held attitude.

A related consistency theory is Festinger's *cognitive dissonance* theory (1957, 1964). This theory postulates that psychological discomfort is caused when a person's own attitudes conflict with each other or with the person's own behaviour. The person will then seek an attitude or behaviour change which will establish cognitive consonance, that is, harmony between attitudes and behaviour. This may entail the person's seeking information selectively to support the justification for a behaviour. For example, a man with coronary artery disease may feel that looking after his health is important, and yet he may like a high-cholesterol diet. This may lead him to attend closely to any news item that seems to cast doubt upon scientific evidence that cholesterol in the diet contributes to artery disease. In this way he can continue to eat the foods he enjoys without having to feel that he is doing the wrong thing for his health. According to Adams and Bromley (1998), when there is dissonance between an individual's beliefs and behaviour, most people are more likely to change the belief than the behaviour – an important challenge to health teachers.

FACTORS AFFECTING COMMUNICATION AND PERSUASION

Communication in nursing care, whether or not it is intended to be persuasive, is influenced by a number of factors, in particular the setting, the nurse, the patient or client, and the message.

The setting

Picture a crowded, noisy room filled with people and smoke. How easy will it be to carry on a conversation in such a room? While the ideal situation would be the calm and quiet of a private room, the reality is that often nurses communicate with patients in their homes where children may be running about and playing, in hospital wards where the corner of the day room may be the only available venue, or in busy accident and emergency departments. However, some aspects of all environments can be considered for control:

- The noise level. As far as possible the setting should be quiet so that the noise is not distracting to the patient. In the home, turn down television sets, ask others in the vicinity to speak quietly, give children a quiet game or task such as reading or jigsaw puzzles. On the other hand, in a busy hospital ward, the general noise level itself may provide a sort of screen for the patient's privacy; if the ward is too quiet, the nurse-patient interaction may be audible to others.

- The presence of others. While a private room is desirable, when one is not available, keep the voice low and make it clear to others in the room that, for a particular period, the nurse's attention is taken up with the one patient only. This can help to avoid interruption.

- The arrangement of furniture. The patient or client should be comfortable, either in a chair or in bed if this is necessary. Furniture should be placed to allow for face-to-face positioning and eye-to-eye contact. Avoid physical barriers between the participants and arrangements that emphasise inequality in the status of the participants in the interaction.

- Other environmental considerations. Other aspects of the environment can enhance or detract from the likelihood of effective interaction. These may include, for example, the lighting, unpleasant smells, potential distractions such as a telephone. In a hospital setting, remember that although it may be a familiar environment to the nurse, it can be alien and perhaps frightening to the patient.

The nurse

As a planned process, therapeutic and persuasive communication is controlled, to a large extent, by the nurse. Therefore, the nurse's skills and knowledge are crucial to the outcome. To develop competence it is necessary to check not just on mastery of the necessary knowledge, but also on personal skills and attitudes before and after each interaction. With experience, this monitoring may be done throughout a communication session. While acquiring communication skills, a simple self-check such as the set of questions in Box 4.2 may be useful.

Attributes of the successful communicator

Empathy, respect for others and warmth have been noted as important characteristics of the successful therapeutic communicator (Gazda et al 1975, 1999). An empathetic nurse seeks to understand the feelings of the patient, to see things as they must appear through his eyes. Empathy is helpful and conducive to developing a therapeutic relationship. The hypothetical conversation in Box 4.3 provides an illustration.

Respecting others is synonymous with valuing and having confidence in them. As a health teacher, the nurse must hold this position sincerely or the patient will not feel willing and able to participate, to make decisions or to act

BOX 4.2	*Self-check on nursing communication skills*

- Was the language I used at the right level?
- Did I meet the other person's needs, or mine?
- Did I adapt messages to verbal and nonverbal cues?
- Did I provide useful written backup material?
- Did I listen?
- Did I use questions well?
- How did I deal with silences?
- Did I accept or reject views that opposed mine?

BOX 4.3	*Using empathy in communication*

Mrs MacDonald is in hospital, having had a hysterectomy three days ago. She is worrying about her four children at home.

Mrs MacD: 'I hope my husband is able to cope with them. They're such lively kids, and they like to get up to mischief.'

Response 1-Nurse: 'Four children can be a handful. I should know, I have six!'

Response 2-Nurse: 'Oh, I'm sure they're all right. There's nothing for you to worry about.'

Response 3-Nurse: 'You sound a bit worried about your husband coping. Four children can be a handful. Has he spoken of how he's getting along at home?'

The first response is not particularly helpful as the nurse does not acknowledge the worry factor and instead turns the focus to herself. The second response is equally unhelpful, as it trivializes Mrs MacDonald's concern and refuses her the opportunity to talk further about what is worrying her. The third response offers the basis for a helpful interaction. The nurse has attended to the content of what Mrs MacDonald has said and acknowledges her concerns and feeling of worry. It provides an opening for further exploration of the problem. Thus the nurse attempts to place herself imaginatively in the patient's shoes.

on them. Carl Rogers (1974) has referred to 'unconditional positive regard'. By this, he means the unconditional acceptance of the person, regardless of what he is in terms of personality, attitudes or behaviour. Being non-judgemental and accepting the person as he is allows the patient to be himself and to self-explore.

Besides having empathy and respect for the patient, the nurse also must develop a warmth which communicates to the patient that the nurse is there to help, wants to help, and cares about him and his situation. Nonverbal communication skills such as making eye contact, appearing relaxed and showing readiness to listen indicate that the nurse has heard both the content and the feeling in what the patient says. Box 4.4 summarizes the points made about empathy, respect and warmth by listing some communication tips.

Credibility can be important, particularly if there is a need to persuade or give advice. Experiments have shown that people are more likely to be per-

BOX 4.4	*Some tips for therapeutic communication*

Do	*Don't*
establish a trusting relationship	be glib
allow the patient the freedom to participate	make premature judgements
be helpful	be opinionated
set up a conducive atmosphere	belittle
regard the information as confidential	change the subject

suaded by a message if the source seems credible to them. To be accepted as credible, the communicator has to be acknowledged as having expertise and being trustworthy and knowledgeable.

In early explorations of the idea of credibility, Hovland and Weiss (1951) demonstrated that the New England Journal of Medicine was more persuasive than a monthly picture magazine in discussing the advisability of selling anti-histamine drugs without prescription. Presumably this is because doctors are regarded as having expert knowledge about drugs, and a professional journal is therefore more persuasive than one generally intended for lay people.

In some instances, credibility depends upon having relevant experience. Levine and Valle (1975) found that former alcoholics were more influential than others in changing students' attitudes about alcoholism, and McPeek and Edwards (1975) demonstrated that long-haired males were more persuasive in arguing against marijuana. This idea has been used in recent advertising campaigns on the topic of HIV and AIDS, with sufferers who failed to practise 'safe sex' or who shared needles to inject drugs giving advice from a position of first-hand experience.

Credibility of source produces attitude change by a process Kelman (1961) has labelled internalization. This means that the new attitude becomes part of the individual's own value or belief system. New information may be resisted if it conflicts with the person's existing value system, or if it causes cognitive dissonance, but once new beliefs are internalized, they tend to be firmly held, even if the source changes stance on the issue. The concept of internalization has since been explored in relation to motivation and attitude change in a wide range of areas (e.g. Proffitt & Kaiser 1998; Barbuto 2000).

Another aspect of source credibility which should be noted is the sleeper effect. This is so called because a number of studies have shown that low-credibility sources appear to increase their impact after a time lapse (Hovland et al 1949; Stiff 1994; Underwood & Pezdek 1998). Why this should be so has not been established, but some researchers have suggested that because the source has low credibility the recipient is more likely to question the original message. Active involvement in producing counter-arguments causes the individual to examine his existing belief system, and convinces him of the validity of the position he initially resisted but eventually adopts.

Attractiveness of the source of a message also influences whether or not it will be well received. People are more likely to adopt attitudes of those they find likeable. Response to source attractiveness is said to happen in order to enhance self-concept. This process Kelman (1961) labelled identification. In this instance the individual will accept the attitude without internalizing it. However, to maintain such an attitude, the influence of the source must be continued. Once the source of influence is removed the attitude may be changed quite readily. In addition, if the communicator's attitude changes, the recipient's will also be likely to change.

Whereas attitude change by internalization usually depends on verification of the information being presented, change by identification is not dependent upon the validity of the position held nor on the existence of evidence to support it. Norman (1976) demonstrated that a communicator was equally persuasive to groups whether or not he presented any reasons supporting the opinion that people sleep more than they need to. The impact of charisma is clearly relevant here.

Source attractiveness would appear to be a somewhat tenuous means of persuasion. Yet widespread use of communicator attractiveness is made in health education, as demonstrated by the use of sports and other media personalities in promoting positive health images. One reason for this is that attractive sources often possess skills and attributes which make them especially persuasive people. Attractive sources may therefore change attitudes by internalization as well as by identification, and this assumption underlies the widespread use of 'celebrities' or image-sellers. It should be remembered that this strategy is also widely used in commercial advertising, which sometimes entails anti-health messages.

Power in the communicator brings about attitude change by a process Kelman (1961) has termed compliance. He proposed that when a communicator has a powerful position with respect to the person receiving the message, there will be a tendency for the recipient to adopt the communicator's position publicly, but reject it privately. Power is exercised by the use of reward or punishment. In nursing settings it is not difficult to imagine that some clients or patients may feel vulnerable and respond to a powerful health care professional by wishing to please or to avoid incurring displeasure. (One doesn't want to be labelled a 'bad patient'!) Power exercised in this way can be very successful in achieving apparent persuasion, but the results are likely to be short-lived once the powerful influence is removed. This may be one explanation of the repeated finding that patients fail to continue with a prescribed medical regimen once they leave hospital.

Psychologists studying persuasion use the word compliance in this quite specific sense. The term compliance is also used widely by health professionals, but here the intended meaning is different and 'compliance' is used to refer to continued adherence to professional health recommendations. Much traditional patient education has been based upon the idea of achieving such adherence, and the use of the word compliance for a successful outcome has not necessarily been an indication that the intention was to bring about change by the exercise of power. Nonetheless, it is important to note the dangers of the exercise of power, as well as its short-lived effects. Today it is no longer universally agreed that patients and clients should accept unquestioningly what health professionals tell them is good for them, and increasingly the emphasis is upon releasing patient power and reducing professional power.

Similarity between sender and receiver can also increase the likelihood that the message will persuade. The explanation for this may be quite simple, in that a similar source appears either credible or attractive or both. If the receiver recognizes the sender as being a kindred type of person, this tends to be perceived as a positive trait.

Credibility, attractiveness, power and similarity are all important characteristics to consider in choosing an effective communicator. Clearly these factors are not always separable in practice; a doctor, for instance, may be a powerful source of communication by virtue of the expertise and trustworthiness which give him credibility, and by the power of his professional position. Nurses, on the other hand, may be attractive sources of communication because they are perceived as less technically educated than doctors and therefore more similar to lay people. On the other hand, while that very feature may in some instances increase credibility because 'the nurse understands, her experience of life is like mine', in other cases it may decrease credibility because 'the nurse understands my position, but does she really know about the medical facts?' So the communicator role is complex and there are no easy or absolute rules. The most satisfying and potentially useful approach to communication is for the nurse to examine what he or she has to bring to the situation, identifying factors which are likely to be strengths and weaknesses in regard to the particular person with whom the communication is to take place, the nature of the message, and the setting in which communication takes place.

The patient or client

There are many features of the person which may affect the communication process. First, his psycho physiological state is important. Can he participate or has he some condition such as deafness, being in a coma, or being in a catatonic state which will severely limit, even totally block, attempts at communication? The nurse's initial assessment of the patient will identify his psycho-physiological state. Factors to note include educational level, age, developmental state and emotions.

Second, what is the patient's perception of the nurse? Is the nurse seen as a helper or as a nuisance? Has the patient had previous experience of health care personnel which now leads him to distrust them? Does the nurse have credibility, attractiveness and power which he acknowledges?

Third, are there sociocultural factors present that the nurse needs to be aware of before helping the patient? For instance, are there religious dietary rules the patient follows which might affect the strict adherence to a specified diet? Even more important, and sometimes difficult to ascertain, is whether there are sociocultural influences which direct the patient's values and attitudes and therefore affect his motivation towards learning new health behaviours.

Fourth, are there personality characteristics which might affect communication? A dependent, chronically anxious person may be unable to self-explore to a depth which would encourage resolution of a problem, whereas a confident person who is used to facing challenges and taking risks may be highly motivated to try new health behaviours.

Two particular aspects of personality have generally been considered to have an effect upon how the individual will respond to persuasive health messages. These are perceived locus of control and self-esteem, which are believed to be inter-related (e.g. Kliewer & Sandler 1992). Some people are more confident than others in their ability to control the environment in which they live. This aspect of personality has been labelled locus of control, or internal-external control. Rotter (1954, 1966, 1975) proposes that people who are at the internal end of the control continuum believe that events occur as a consequence of their own actions and under their control. Those at the external end, on the other hand, believe that events are not related to their personal behaviour and are therefore beyond their control (Adams & Bromley 1998).

Since persuasive communication is usually directed at the individual from an external source, it seems likely that persons who see themselves as in control of the environment will be less likely to be influenced by external factors, and will therefore resist persuasion rather well. There is some substance to this idea, but equally, it is possible that people who do not see themselves as being in control see no point in any health-related action, since, after all, most things are outside their personal control.

Everyone holds a concept of self. Some people see themselves in a favourable light, others less so. This evaluative aspect of self-concept is called self-esteem. Carl Rogers (1951, 1959) claimed that a favourable self-concept is a necessary condition for mental health. Knowing that other people think well of them seems important to most people. Psychologists have proposed that the seeking of positive comments from others motivates and directs human behaviour. Health educators utilizing an educational model have attempted to capitalize on this phenomenon by designing educational programmes intended to promote self-esteem. The recent 'Be All You Can Be' health education campaign in Scotland exemplified this approach.

There is a clear case within nursing for promoting self-esteem in patients and in clients. It is less clear, however, what part self-esteem plays in governing responses to persuasion. It and other aspects of personality appear to be interlinked with social, psychological and cultural factors in determining health-related behaviour.

The message

While this aspect of communication may seem straightforward, researchers have discovered that messages may have complex repercussions. The nature and content of the message, as well as the style of presentation, affect the way in which the message is processed by the recipient and the extent to which it will persuade. Some factors of note in persuasive messages are:

One-sided versus two-sided arguments

Research has been done on whether people are more easily persuaded if the message presents one or two sides of an argument. Hovland et al (1949) demonstrated that two-sided messages were more effective with better educated audiences, while less well educated people were more easily persuaded by one-sided messages. In practice, of course, what happens in laboratory-type conditions is of doubtful relevance to the health educator, since it is unlikely that any intended recipient can be kept free of contamination by other views in today's world. Sooner or later the health educator who presents only one side of a case will be discredited. Despite this obvious truth, there is often a tendency for professionals to attempt to package information in a simplistic message that contains only part of the truth, or just one view on it, when communicating with people whom they perceive to be uneducated. It is likely that the mere presenting of two sides to an argument is less significant than the quality of the case presented and its relevance to the intended audience (Severin & Tankard 2001).

Repetition

There is evidence that repetition of a message is in itself persuasive. Greater exposure to a message has been found to increase recall and attitude formation (Solomon 1972). Advertisers take message exposure to saturation level, sometimes even repeating the same message twice during the same break between television programmes. However, the exact mechanism by which repetition operates is not known, and at times repetition is tiresome and can generate negative reactions. What evidence there is suggests that the greatest benefits of repetition will accrue where the message is complex, and that repetition of simple messages, with the risk of 'overkill', can be counterproductive and should be avoided. In addition, in at least one research study, it has been shown that repetition does not necessarily have a positive effect in clinical populations (Chiaravalloti et al 2003).

Fear arousal

A number of researchers have looked at whether fear will motivate people to take preventive action in relation to their health. Use of fear arousal as a health education technique is suggested on the grounds that people will be motivated to reduce the risk of developing a particular disease if they are presented with fear-producing information about the condition while at the same time being given reassuring advice about how to avoid it. For instance, in a recent British television health promotion campaign, actors playing the role of cancer patients in the last stages of their disease make a plea to viewers to stop smoking.

Janis and Fesbach (1953) demonstrated that high fear appeals work less well than low fear appeals in motivating people to adopt good dental hygiene practices. That finding cast doubt on the use of fear arousal as a health education technique. Later studies, however, have shown that fear arousal may be effective in some circumstances.

Leventhal (1970) has provided a possible explanation of why the response to fear appeals varies. He proposed that fear arousal is likely to provoke two parallel responses in the individual: fear control and danger control. Individuals receiving fear-arousing messages will be motivated to control fear as well as danger. In some circumstances, particularly in high threat, the need to control fear would outweigh the need to control danger, and emotional response might just prevent the person from taking any action against the disease. It is possible, for instance, that fear arousal in breast cancer education might result in a woman's being afraid to find out she has the disease, making her too afraid to present herself for mammography.

Two studies supported this proposition by demonstrating that those who perceive themselves as being at risk are less likely to be influenced to action by high fear appeals. Leventhal and Watts (1966) demonstrated this in regard to smokers' response to communication about lung cancer, and Berkowitz and Cottingham (1966) showed that fear appeals in relation to seat belt use were less effective with regular than occasional drivers. It seems that people who see themselves as vulnerable respond by controlling fear and the fear–control response inhibits action to control the danger.

It is also possible that people with high self-esteem respond to fear appeals while people with low self-esteem do not. A study by Goldstein (1959) showed that people labelled as 'copers', confronted with a high fear arousal message and a specific plan of avoiding action, adopted the recommended action, while those identified as 'avoiders' did not.

In general, it can be said that fear appeals work with some people and in some circumstances, but that it is difficult to predict the effects of arousing fear. Further, as Sarafino (1990) points out, messages need to contain specific advice for preventive action and strategies to promote confidence, so the mere generation of fear cannot be expected to be effective in motivating a change in behaviour.

Message content

It is difficult to locate research in the area of message content. Fishbein and Ajzen (1981) identified this as a serious omission, asserting that message content interacts with other factors in accomplishing persuasion. They argued that indirect effects of the message, in other words, the impact upon beliefs other than the ones to which the message is addressed, should be given special consideration when messages are designed. For instance, an advertising claim that a detergent is powerful may cause housewives to react favourably to it because a powerful detergent may be expected to get the wash clean. However, some housewives may believe that powerful detergents harm clothes and this may generate a negative reaction to the message.

Impact effects are clearly of importance in health teaching. Consider the impact on pregnant females who are smokers of the fact that smoking during pregnancy reduces birth weight: if they believe that low birth weight will be an advantage in labour, or that small babies are more attractive than heavy ones, then they are not likely to be discouraged from smoking. Fishbein and Ajzen also argued that there is little to gain from manipulating factors that will increase attention to or understanding of the message, since some messages seem to be accepted without any supporting evidence: people do adopt new ideas without any detailed understanding of why they matter. This, however, seems more likely to be a consideration for the pure researcher or the propagandist than for the nurse as health teacher.

The interrelationship of sender–receiver message factors

It is evident that there are as many questions as answers arising from research in the field of persuasive communication. However, review of theories and research studies suggests that the message is more likely to persuade if the conditions indicated in Figure 4.7 are met. What individual studies fail to illuminate is whether or how such factors are interrelated.

In persuasive communication, the central question of what motivates the health-related actions of an individual remains. Rosenstock (1974) records that early research attempts to explain why individuals take or avoid preventive health action led to the development of the Health Belief Model. The original model proposed that the combined effect of an individual's perception of

ACTIVITY 4.2

One evening, watch a television news or current affairs programme in which politicians participate, and spend two hours of the evening watching a commercial channel. As you watch, be alert for instances of intended persuasion and make brief notes on them. Analyse these incidents in relation to the factors highlighted in this chapter. For example, consider the following questions (and you will probably think of others):

■ Who is trying to persuade, who are they trying to persuade, and why?

■ What is the content of the message the persuader is trying to impart?

■ What features of the persuader and/or the message enhance or detract from the likelihood of successful persuasion?

■ Who among viewers would be likely to be persuaded, and who would not?

■ How do issues such as fear, beliefs, etc., come into it?

■ Finally, of the instances you observed, which persuaded you? Why? Did any have the opposite effect? Why?

| FIGURE 4.7 | *Conditions for effective persuasion* |

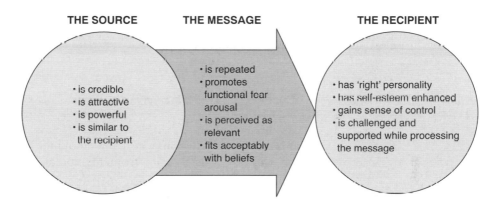

the severity of a disease and his own susceptibility to it would provide the energy or force to act to prevent the disease, provided he was sufficiently convinced that the prescribed course of action would be beneficial and worth his personal trouble and costs.

Becker (1974) has provided a collection of papers which record how the Health Belief Model was tested and developed. The model posed questions about the role of beliefs about susceptibility, seriousness and perceived benefits in motivating preventive health actions. It then provided for examination of ways in which factors such as age, sex, race, ethnicity, personality, social class, peer pressure and knowledge from various sources would interrelate to increase or decrease the likelihood of the individual's taking preventive health action.

Rosenstock et al (1988, 1994) suggest that there are key variables that need to be taken into consideration when applying the Health Belief Model to health issues such as HIV/AIDS. These are:

- the perceived threat (relating to both the perceived susceptibility of the person and the perceived severity of the health problem)
- the perceived benefits of adopting the recommended advice
- the perceived barriers or negative consequences
- cues that will motivate action
- other relevant variables (e.g. demographic, social, psychological, structural)
- self-efficacy.

In commenting on the state of research related to the role of beliefs in motivating health actions, Kirscht (1974) has suggested that the various trials of the Health Belief Model do substantiate the idea that beliefs energize and direct behaviour. What is not as clear, however, is which set of beliefs is sufficient to predict or direct any given behaviour, and what processes enter into belief change in relation to behaviour. Despite all the work that has been done, research on modifying beliefs and behaviour still leaves much to be done.

In the circumstances, the best the practising health educator can do is provide a check list of possible beliefs and the psychosocial and cultural factors which seem likely to militate for or against the proposed action by the person, and keep these in mind when assessing teaching needs. The application of this approach is demonstrated in Chapter 6.

REFERENCES

Adams B, Bromley B 1998 Psychology for Health Care – Key Terms and Concepts. Macmillan, Basingstoke.

Azen I, Fishbein M 1977 Attitude-behaviour relations: a theoretical analysis and review of empirical research. Psychological Bulletin 84: 888-918.

Barbuto JE 2000 Identifying the sources of motivation in the post-game press conference: an exercise for applying an integrative taxonomy of motivation. Journal of Behavioral and Applied Management 4(1): 41-50.

Becker MH (ed) 1974 The health belief model and personal health behaviour. Slack, Thorofare New Jersey.

Berkowitz L, Cottingham DR 1966 The interest value and relevance of fear arousing communications. Journal of Abnormal and Social Psychology 60: 37-43.

Blaxter M 1990 Health & lifestyles.

Tavistock/Routledge, London.

Burton G & Dimbleby R 1995 Between Ourselves, 2nd edn. Edward Arnold, London.

Chiaravalloti N D, Demaree H, Gaudino EA, DeLuca J 2003 Can repetition effect maximize learning in multiple sclerosis? Clinical rehabilitation 17(1): 58-68.

Festinger L 1957 A theory of cognitive dissonance. Stanford University Press, Stanford California.

Festinger L 1964 Conflict decision and dissonance. Stanford University Press, Stanford California.

Fishbein M, Ajzen I 1981 Acceptance yielding and impact: cognitive processes in persuasion. In: Petty RE, Ostram TM, Brock TC (eds) Cognitive responses in persuasion. Lawrence Erlbaum, Hillsdale New Jersey.

Garrett A 1972 Interviewing, its principles and methods, 2nd edn. Family Service

Association of America, New York.

Gazda GM, Asbury FR, Balzer FJ, Childers WC, Phelps RE, Walters RP 1999 Human Relations Development: A manual for educators, 6th edn. Allyn & Bacon, Boston.

Gazda GM, Walters RP, Childers WC 1975 Human relations development: a manual for health sciences. Allyn & Bacon, London.

Goldstein M 1959 The relationship between coping and avoiding behaviour and response to fear arousing propaganda. Journal of Abnormal and Social Psychology 58: 247-252.

Hanson E 1996 Stress and the person with cancer: an exploration of the concept of the stress and the nurse's psychological support role. In: Soothill K, Henry C, Kendrick K, Themes and Perspectives in Nursing, 2nd edn. Chapman & Hall, London.

Hovland CI, Lumsdaine A, Sheffield FD 1949 Experiments on mass communication. Princeton University Press, Princeton, New Jersey.

Hovland CI, Weiss W 1951 The influence of source credibility on communication effectiveness. Public Opinion Quarterly 15: 635-650.

Janis IL, Fesbach S 1953 Effects of fear arousing communications. Journal of Abnormal and Social Psychology 48: 78-92.

Katz D 1960 The functional approach to the study of attitudes. Public Opinion Quarterly 24: 163-204.

Kelman H 1961 Processes of opinion change. Public Opinion Quarterly 25: 57-58.

Kirsht JP 1974 Research related to the modification of health beliefs. In: Becker MH (ed) The health belief model and personal health behaviour. Slack, Thorofare New Jersey.

Kliewer W, Sandler IN 1992 Locus of control and self-esteem as moderators of stress-symptom relations in children and adolescents. Journal of Abnormal Child Psychology 20, 393-413.

La Piere RT 1934 Attitudes versus actions. Social Forces 13: 230-237.

Leventhal H 1970 Findings and theory in the study of fear communications. In: Berkowitz L (ed) Advances in experimental social psychology 5. Academic Press, New York.

Leventhal H, Watts JC 1966 Sources of resistance to fear arousing communications on smoking and lung cancer. Journal of Personality 34: 155-175.

Levine IM, Valle R 1975 The convert as a credible source. Social Behaviour and Personality 3(1): 81.

McPeek RW, Edwards JD 1975 Expectancy, disconfirmation and attitude change. Journal of Social Psychology 96(2): 193-207.

Norman R 1976 When what is said is important: a comparison of expert and attractive sources. Journal of Experimental Psychology 12: 294-300.

Osgood CE, Tannenbaum PH 1955 The principle of congruity in the prediction of attitude change. Psychological Review 62: 42-55.

Osgood CE, Suci GJ, Tannenbaum PH 1957 The measurement of meaning. University of Illinois Press, Urbana, Illinois.

Petty RE, Ostram TM, Brock TC (eds) 1981 Cognitive responses in persuasion. Lawrence Erlbaum Associates, Hillsdale, New Jersey.

Proffitt DR, Kaiser MK 1998 The internalization of perceptual processing of constraints. In: Hochberg J (Ed.) Perception and cognition at century's end (pp. 169-197). Academic Press, San Diego, CA, USA.

Rogers CR 1951 Client centred therapy: its current practice implications and theory. Houghton Mifflin, Boston.

Rogers CR 1959 A theory of therapy personality and interpersonal relationships as developed in a client centred framework. In: Koch S (ed) Psychology: a study of science, vol 3. McGraw Hill, New York.

Rogers C 1974 On becoming a person, 4th edn. Constable, London.

Rosenstock IM 1974 Historical origins of the health belief model. In: Becker MH (ed) The health belief model and personal health behaviour. Slack, Thorofare New Jersey.

Rosenstock IM, Strecher VJ, Becker MH. 1988 Social learning theory and the health belief model. Health Education Quarterly 15, 175-183.

Rosenstock IM, Strecher VJ, Becker MH 1994 The Health Belief Model and HIV risk behaviour change. In Peterson J, DiClemente R (eds) Preventing AIDS: Theory and Practice of Behavioral Interventions. Plenum Press, New York, pp 5-24.

Rotter JB 1954 Social learning and clinical psychology. Prentice Hall, Englewood Cliffs New Jersey.

Rotter JB 1966 Generalised expectations for internal versus external control of reinforcement. Psychological Monographs 80(1): 1-28.

Rotter JB 1975 Some problems and misconceptions related to the construct of internal versus external control of reinforcement. Journal of Consulting and

Clinical Psychology 43, 56-67.

Sarafino E 1990 Health psychology: biopsychosocial interactions. John Wiley & Sons, New York

Severin WJ, Tankard JW 2001 Communication Theories, 5th edn. Allyn & Bacon.

Solomon H 1972 The effects of multiple exposure source credibility and initial option on communication effectiveness.

Dissertation Abstracts International 33(3-A): 1227.

Stiff JB 1994 Persuasive communication. Guilford, New York.

Underwood J, Pezdek K 1998 Memory suggestibility as an example of the sleeper effect. Psychonomic Bulletin & Review 5, 449-453.

5 | Teaching techniques and aids

One of the tasks of the health teacher is to present information effectively. Being able to do this depends on selecting teaching strategies and aids that will encourage and stimulate understanding and retention.

TEACHING FOR UNDERSTANDING AND RECALL

It is basic to cognitive learning that the learner be able to comprehend the message or information that needs to be understood. One of the main barriers to communication between professionals and lay people is that many people are unfamiliar with the *technical language* that nurses and doctors use every day. There are two ways to tackle the problem. Sometimes lay terms can be substituted for technical ones, thus setting the person at ease. Having a familiar starting point facilitates the absorption of new material. The other approach is to use the technical term and to explain its meaning. Generally this is more useful because it may help the person in future communications with other health care professionals, and it helps to avoid giving the impression of talking down to the person. Access to technical language can be an asset to patients, helping them to achieve partnership in communication.

A study of communication between general practitioners and patients (Pratt et al 1957) demonstrated that people without a facility for technical language can be at a disadvantage. Eighty-nine general practitioners were observed communicating with 214 patients. All the doctors tended to underestimate the patients' knowledge. Those they perceived as particularly poorly informed were given less information than those the doctors thought were quite well informed. A curious vicious circle was observed. The doctor arbitrarily assessed a given patient and assumed he would have little or no technical language. The doctor then avoided using such language during the consultation and made no attempt to deal with any complex issues because of his conviction that the patient would not understand in any case. In turn, the patient, sensitive to a lack of information being offered by the doctor, responded by not asking any questions. Although this study is now quite old, the insights it offers are still current. A research team in Canada is currently working on a study which should add useful understandings about patient-professional communication with a particular focus on cancer patients once it is completed in 2004 (Thorne et al 2002).

When talking to people about health, the professional health teacher should avoid using jargon that may alienate. Nonetheless, using and explaining technical terms may be helpful in reducing people's dependency on health care professionals. In general, younger and more educated people will understand more technical language, but such assumptions should be avoided, in both directions. That is, one should not assume either a high or low level of prior knowledge. It is best to discover what each individual's starting point is. It is always best to ask the person what things mean to him, since sometimes lay and professional people use the same terms but with different meanings.

It is also worthwhile to remember that there is a limit to everyone's memory, thus the *amount of information* to be given must be considered carefully. It is important in health teaching to present only as much information as people can cope with at one time. It is often better to deliver small packages of information in several sessions, rather than trying to cover a great deal within one or two sessions.

The *sequencing* of items of information also has an impact on recall and understanding. To achieve effective understanding, information needs to be presented in a logical sequence. In addition, people generally find it easiest to remember the first part of what is said, so the health teacher should introduce important aspects of information early in the presentation.

People also remember best those things they perceive as being important to them. A study by Ley and Spelman (1965) showed that hospital outpatients remembered information about their diagnosis and illness better than they remembered information about investigations or instructions for care. This is understandable, as people are naturally anxious about what is wrong with them. The health teacher should be aware of this, and should attend to it, and allow the person time to come to terms with it, before trying to impart detailed information the person will need to remember about how to manage his or her self-care.

It is also important for the health teacher to *structure* the information. Most people will remember information more easily if they are able to fit it into their own mental constructions. This enables them to understand it (deep learning) rather than just memorizing it (surface learning). It means that it is important for the teacher to find out what the learner's current level of knowledge is before trying to teach. During the presentation, it may help for the health teacher to categorize the information and indicate the number of items in each category. For instance, the nurse might structure a message to a hospital patient in this way: 'I am going to tell you about your diagnosis, the results of the investigations done while you have been in hospital, and about your treatment. Firstly, about your diagnosis there are two things to say ...', and so on.

Often when advice is not followed or is forgotten, the reason is that its presentation has been insufficiently *specific*. An instruction to 'take it easy', for example, is too vague to have real meaning. What would be slowing down for some people would represent increased activity for others. General statements are neither convincing nor helpful, and people forget what they find difficult to interpret. This is equally true for information that is given in a form other than in-person presentation. A series of experiments described by Ley (1976) showed that improved readability together with categorization of information items and specificity can increase the effectiveness of a patient education leaflet. In one of these experiments, leaflets were used to assist people to lose weight. It was found that an experimental group exposed to a specifically designed leaflet lost considerably more weight than a control group exposed to a standard leaflet.

The use of *written material* can be useful as a reminder of information that has been taught, and it gives the person more control over the pace at which the information is processed. It is important that such written material is well structured and clear. With detailed information or information that may be difficult to understand, it is useful to include diagrams. The language used should be easily understood and readable. For example, Meade (1988), in a study on people's comprehension of smoking literature, showed that adjusting the level of reading ability required for the written material had an impact on how readily the information was comprehended. Readability can be enhanced by the use of short sentences and words with few syllables, when this is possible, though it should not be to the extent of talking down to the reader. Written material is likely to be more effective if it is attractively presented, so attention should be given to the layout and visual impact of the material.

In some cases, it may be appropriate to involve the patient in preparing the written material, which may be in the form of notes that relate to the individual circumstances. Things are generally remembered and understood better if the learner participates actively in the learning event (Dean & Kenworthy 2000; Davis 1993).

The *immediate personal experience* of the patient, factors such as anxiety or pain, may impair his or her usual ability to understand or recall information. Important instructions should therefore be timed carefully and repeated as necessary. For example, though it may be helpful to outline postoperative care preoperatively, it is unrealistic to expect anyone to remember details at a time of high anxiety. Clearly, it will be necessary to repeat some information. It may even be helpful to withhold unnecessary detail of postoperative progress until after surgery has taken place. Similarly, someone in acute pain immediately after admission with myocardial infarction should not be subjected to any more detail than is necessary.

It is not always easy to judge how much information patients want or can cope with, and when is the best time to give it. Some people, even in considerable pain or distress, will indicate that they want to know what is likely to happen to them and what treatments will be undertaken. Information should not be withheld, though many people may be satisfied initially with brief answers if they are assured that an opportunity to discuss detail will follow. That assurance will not be provided by evasiveness and a vague promise to tell later, but rather by an obvious willingness to listen and to supply information as and when the person indicates a desire for it.

All of these factors – the use of technical language, the amount of information and its sequence, organization and specificity, the use of written reminders and consideration of the immediate personal experience of the learner – are important considerations when trying to increase understanding and recall.

TEACHING FOR SKILLS LEARNING

When patients or clients need to learn how to do something, it is obvious that learning information will not be sufficient, though it is likely to be necessary to underpin action. As mentioned earlier, learning is generally more effective when the learner is active in the process, and this is particularly true for psychomotor skills. Thus it is important, in order to learn to perform a skill, that the learner is able to observe it and practise it, and then receive feedback about the practice. The learner will also need the opportunity to ask questions. Details about the use of demonstration in teaching are covered later in this chapter.

ENCOURAGING AFFECTIVE LEARNING

Teaching for affective learning is in some respects more difficult than teaching for the other two domains. For one thing, the teacher needs to be aware of the difference between teaching and indoctrinating. Topics that relate to attitudes and beliefs inevitably have implications for the individual's right to make decisions about his or her own life. Thus there is a fine balance to be struck, and the health professional involved in such teaching needs to be alert to the ethics of the situation.

Since much affective learning touches on feelings and beliefs, it may be most effectively addressed in a context that involves the learner in active participation. The learner needs the opportunity to question and evaluate, to express feelings, to argue and explore. For this to be successful, it is important for the teacher to establish a climate that is open and non-judgemental so the learner will feel comfortable about participating. The sections about group work and role play later in this chapter are particularly relevant for affective learning.

TEACHING METHODS

The lecture method

Much teaching necessitates the presentation of information. Nurses often do this with patients or clients on an individual basis, but sometimes a number of people need to be taught the same things. In such cases nurses may give lectures or talks to groups. The lecture is a traditional teaching technique that offers a useful way of presenting learners with a framework of what is to be learned.

Format and use of the lecture

In health teaching, a lecture should usually be quite short, probably just 15 or 20 minutes, and it should be well organized with a clear-cut beginning and end. The usual order of proceedings is to introduce oneself, if necessary, and clarify the object of the lecture, give a brief outline of the content and describe the format of the session, give the lecture, summarize the session, and thank the learners for their attention. In some situations it may be helpful to give a handout as a printed reminder of what has been said.

The lecture can be combined with other methods. For example, a series of sessions on preparation for childbirth might be introduced with a short lecture, with the later sessions being practical and active on the part of the learners. A short talk is often a very welcome beginning to a new course as not everyone will want to plunge into discussion or participation straight away. An introductory outline of material will often alert listeners to items they may raise in discussion later. Despite changes in teaching methods in schools, there is still widespread acceptance of the idea that in a teaching session the teacher will do the talking. While it will be useful to establish later that all group members have a role to play in exploring health issues, having the teacher speak first is often a reassuring beginning as this is a procedure familiar to most people.

Delivery. Delivery of the lecture is very much a matter of personal style; some mannerisms add to the speaker's attractiveness, others detract. There are a number of 'dos and don'ts' that are useful to keep in mind: do move while lecturing but don't pace; do make eye contact with everyone in the audience; don't use 'um' or 'er' frequently; do be well prepared so as to avoid embarrassing pauses, but don't feel you must be speaking all the time – people may need thinking time or may like to take notes; and don't overuse or 'speak to' the blackboard or projecting screen, otherwise the learners will view mostly the lecturer's back. Visual material should be clear, easy to read and attractively presented.

Using notes can help the teacher maintain a cogent argument and prevent too many irrelevant anecdotes, but on the other hand, it is important to maintain a lively delivery and make contact with the audience, so reading verbatim from notes should be avoided. It may be best to use annotated headings rather than a detailed script. The lecture should be given within the allotted time, which means keeping an eye on a watch or clock. Beyond the scheduled time the listeners' attention will begin to wander. Early in the presentation, the teacher should check that his or her voice can be heard.

Limitations. It is wise to remember that a lecture presents the information in the same manner to all those who are listening, whatever their needs. Since people process information differently and absorb new information at varying paces, some people may learn very little. The lecture method, therefore, has limitations in health teaching and should not be the only method of choice if the intention is to help people explore ideas and examine attitudes. Keeping the initial talk to 20 minutes or less and following it with an opportunity for questions can help to overcome some of the method's shortcomings. Alternatively, when a teaching session is to last an hour or so, it may be possible to arrange for material to be presented in three short episodes interspersed with opportunities for the group to ask questions and discuss. Again, this is a good way to begin a series of lessons because the initial questions and discussion can help the teacher to appraise the level of knowledge and type of teaching required and thus to make immediate adjustments to suit the learners' needs.

It will be necessary to have a strategy for coping with the silence which almost inevitably falls when the first opportunity to ask questions is given. There are two common reasons for silence. The first is that people need time to formulate questions. It is important to relax and wait and so make time available; there is always a temptation to dash in with something to fill the void. In health teaching this is particularly counterproductive because nurses are often asked to teach people with whom they have relatively limited contact, and questions may be the best clue available to the real learning needs.

The second reason for the initial silence may be that the majority of people in the group find it difficult to ask questions. They may be afraid to expose ignorance, have little experience of speaking up in a group of people, or consider that questioning may be interpreted as showing ignorance or challenging the teacher's authority. Again, this can be overcome by waiting in a relaxed manner and by reducing any threat in the way the question is asked. The bold 'Are there any questions?' may be substituted by, 'I'll stop now and give you a chance to say something ...' or such prompts as, 'Have any of you had the experience of ...?', 'What do you think of this (picture, idea, etc.)?' and so on. The first question or comment from the group may open the gate to a flood of others. Questions should be responded to positively as this invites further risk-taking on the part of the listeners. Starting a reply by saying something like 'I'm glad you asked that' or 'That brings up an interesting point' acknowledges and appreciates the participation.

The lecture method of teaching is best suited to the transmission of information, that is, for learning within the cognitive domain. Pure lecture may foster surface-level learning, unless is it modified to allow time for questions or discussion, or used within a programme of sessions which include more participative methods. Elements of psychomotor and affective learning can be addressed within a lecture, in the sense that information about them can be given, but the lecture on its own will not be sufficient for learning in these two domains.

Group work

Grouping people to listen to a lecture, even when they have maximum opportunity to ask questions, is not what is meant by group teaching. Nor is a group automatically formed because the number of people present is small or because seating has been arranged in a circle or semicircle instead of in rows facing front.

Effective group work requires several persons to work and learn together. The presence of other group members and their contributions helps the individual to consider and respond to the feelings, ideas and opinions of others. Group work promotes recognition of similarities and differences. The individual can learn how to participate in the group, thereby increasing interaction skills.

Group work in health teaching depends on the assumption that a group has certain basic characteristics that will facilitate expression of feelings, sharing of ideas and exploration of attitudes and beliefs. In some professional settings, such as social work and psychiatry, group work is used as a therapeutic tool. In health teaching, group work is used as an educational tool and the health educator will often neither have nor exercise the skills of a therapist with respect to the exploration of values and feelings. There is an obvious exception to this in the case of psychiatric nursing, but that is beyond the scope of this text.

Group characteristics

Groups have a number of common characteristics:

- *Definable membership*. A group will have at least two members and they will be distinguished by sharing a common characteristic or type. For instance, a class of student nurses, a group of prenatal mothers, the men sharing a small ward in a cardiac unit, and individuals attending a self-help organization such as Alcoholics Anonymous are all groups.

- *Common identity*. Members of a group have a sense of belonging to the group, whether on a long-term or transient basis; they consciously identify with one another.

- *Interdependence and common goals*. A gathering of people arrives at group feeling when they have the same goals or ideals and when they know they depend on each other to achieve those goals or meet needs. For example, people in pressure groups need each other because collective action will achieve their ends. They associate willingly because they share the same aspirations for change. Likewise, in self-help groups people are conscious that the help of others will assist them to meet their needs, such as for support while stopping smoking.

- *Interaction*. When a group has formed, the members communicate with one another; they respond to the views of others and are influenced by others in the group.

- *Working as one*. In some indefinable way, a group, once formed, takes on its own life and energy. Individuals in the group learn to make their contribution in a way that enables the group to work together, so that the group somehow behaves as a single organism.

Obviously there are many different kinds of groups, more than ever in today's society, but all of them will display, to a greater or lesser extent, these basic characteristics.

Use of groups in health teaching

Nurses will operate as health teachers with two types of group: those whose primary purpose is something other than health learning, such as a Women's Guild, school class, or Parent–Teacher Association; and those especially convened for the purpose of learning about health, such as patients receiving preoperative teaching, groups learning parenting skills, members of the public who have responded to an advertisement offering help to stop smoking, or a group addressing problems related to alcoholism. In either case, group work is used because the process of working in a group has something to offer those who need to learn about their health.

The origins of the use of groups in health education lie in experimental work done in the 1940s by Lewin (1947) who used group process to assist in such activities as motivating women to introduce offal to the family diet or to give babies orange juice. Lewin demonstrated that the group provided a per-suasive force. Housewives in his studies were more persuaded to change by group sessions than by lectures because there was discussion of the problems involved in the change. Having to make and announce a decision and being able to see what other people had decided were also persuasive factors. Generally speaking, individuals are motivated to conform to a group decision to the extent that they need the approval and acceptance of the group.

Use of groups within health teaching has grown as ideas about health edu-cation and health promotion options have developed. Nowadays, health teach-ers still use groups to persuade people to change attitudes. Equally, group work is used to reduce the authority dependence generated by traditional health education approaches, and groups may be set up on an entirely self-directed model on the assumption that the health educator's role is to enable rather than to persuade. Group work can be established either formally or informally (Davis 1993). An example of a formal group would be a school class on sexual health (e.g. Dean 2001), and an example of an informal group on the same topic is suggested in the SPW website (SPW 2003). The formal example refers to a programme consisting of 21 classes per week within the school curriculum of primary and secondary schools in Zimbabwe. The infor-mal example relates to lessons run outside the school curriculum after school hours, also in Zimbabwe. In both cases, there is a strong focus on AIDS awareness and related issues, as Zimbabwe has one of the highest HIV/AIDS rates in the world (Dean 2001).

Preparing for group work

A number of factors that can influence the dynamics of group work should be considered in the planning of group work for health teaching.

Background. If the group is a new one, people will have to get to know each other and find ways of working together. If members are similar to one anoth-er with respect to abilities, attitudes and aptitudes as well as social status, group work will usually be enhanced.

The established existence of a group means that the members may have no need to clarify the task before them. They will already have ways of working together and these may assist the health teaching process. Others may have developed habits that hinder; for instance, some groups have an ingrained hier-archy, some are used to having only a few dominant people speak up, some may argue a lot.

Expectations. If the group has been constituted by the health teacher for the purpose, expectations will be influenced by the advance information given by the health teacher. Groups who invite outside experts such as nurses to teach them have a variety of expectations. Some will want to participate in group work, others may anticipate receiving a lecture. Sometimes the group has exist-ing behavioural constraints which make establishing group work very difficult. People who are used to the teacher doing all the leading and talking and hav-ing all the ideas may find it threatening to be expected to participate.

Size. The ideal size for a group depends on its purpose. In a small group, there is a better chance of gaining participation by all members, and consensus will be more easily achieved. On the other hand, small groups tend to be more expensive of time and resources, and more people can be reached in less time in larger groups. In addition, more ideas may be generated from within a larger group which may lead to the task being accomplished more efficiently. An intermediate size of 10 or 12 members should draw on the positive aspects of both small and large groups and encourage discussion without threat. If it is necessary to deal with a larger group when the task would be better suited to a small group, the whole group may be broken into smaller working groups, or 'buzz groups', for part of the time.

Cohesiveness. While it is important that the group members feel close, if they are too closely knit, this aspect may become dysfunctional. The group needs to be open to new information and ideas. Cooperation and open communication promote a healthy level of cohesiveness.

Environment. Groups generally benefit from feeling that they have a defined place in which to meet. If all goes well in a group then the members will arrange the environment to suit themselves. For the first meeting, however, it may help for the teacher or leader to arrange chairs so people can see and hear each other and to minimize distractions, such as noise, from outside. Physical arrangements need to be reasonably good, but the most important environmental factor is the creation of a relaxed and friendly atmosphere in which people will learn to trust and respect each other.

Formation and function. As a group forms and functions, it may be observed going through a series of stages (see Figure 5.1). Note that, while these stages are numbered sequentially, there are group situations when it is appropriate for the process to recommence. It might be more helpful to think of such an instance as a spiral rather than a cycle, since group members would already be acquainted with one another, so some aspects of the individual phases would be modified a second or third time round.

FIGURE 5.1   *Four stages of group work*

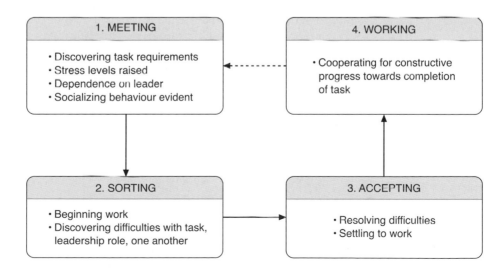

Group roles

In any group the roles assumed by both the leaders and the members are of paramount importance because they may influence the achievement of goals and objectives for each individual within the group and for the group as a whole.

Leadership roles. There is no set of functions that would be universally acknowledged to constitute the leader's role. It varies with the nature and purpose of the group. However, the group usually does have expectations of the leader and the style associated with that role. The style of leadership affects group process. There are teachers who want to maintain control and have the group do things their way at all times. Others allow members to share equally in deciding how to proceed and thus their involvement is equal to that of any other member. Still others allow students to 'do their own thing'. Whichever style is used, the effects on the work of the group should be attended to and evaluated.

Some now classic experiments on the effects of leadership style (White & Lippett 1968) attempted to measure the effects of three different types of leadership behaviour: authoritarian, democratic and laissez-faire. Results showed that *authoritarian leadership*, where the leader took complete control of the group, increased the quantity and quality of work that the group could produce in the short term. However, group members demonstrated hostility to each other and to the leader, and there was aggression and competition. In addition, groups led by authoritarian leaders were more discontented, developed dependence on the leader and showed less originality. Groups working under *democratic leadership*, where the leader kept some control of the group but encouraged involvement of members in making decisions, were much slower in producing work. They appeared to be more motivated, however, and their productivity increased as time went on. The atmosphere in these groups was friendly; members praised each other's efforts, worked as a team and were satisfied with the arrangements for the group. Under *laissez-faire leadership*, where the leader remained in the background and allowed group members to take all the initiative, less work was done and it was of poorer quality. Members were aggressive and wasted time more than in the other groups.

Clearly, for some groups, authoritarian leadership may be best, especially if there is a specific task to be completed in a short time. Generally speaking, however, the democratic style of leadership is more likely to be useful in health teaching, since the aim is to increase independence in those being taught. Laissez-faire leadership is generally considered to be the least effective style, but it may nevertheless be appropriate in some situations. For example, if a health professional has been asked to do an informal session with a self-help group, it may be appropriate to 'lead' the session with a very light touch and let the participants steer it according to their perceived needs. It should be pointed out that these three leadership styles are 'ideal types' – that is, they are pure in the idea of them, but they are not necessarily pure in the real world, and often the leadership style that is exercised is a mixture. In some instances it is useful for the health teacher to adopt different leadership styles at different points in the proceedings.

Member roles. Early work on group roles (Benne & Sheats 1948) distinguished functions in relation, first, to group building and maintenance and,

BOX 5.1	*Group roles* Benne & Sheats 1948

Building and maintenance functions

- Encouraging – being friendly, responsive, praising, accepting contributions
- Mediating – conciliating, compromising
- Gate-keeping – facilitating contributions by others
- Following – being an audience, a good listener
- Relieving tension – draining off negative feelings by joking or clarifying the subject

Group task functions

- Introducing new ways of looking at things
- Information seeking and giving
- Opinion giving
- Clarifying
- Elaborating
- Summarizing

second, to group tasks. These are shown in Box 5.1. On the breakdown as detailed, it is obvious that leadership and membership roles may be inter-changeable.

Potential problems

In any group, problems may arise. Many of these are related to self-centred behaviour of members. The following may need to be dealt with from time to time, either by the leader or by the group:

- *Obstructive moves that block progress.* These may include going off on a tangent, rejecting ideas without consideration, or arguing on a point everyone else has accepted. Obstructive members may withdraw from the activity by using deliberate silence or behaviour that indicates lack of interest (e.g. yawning, talking to neighbours, doodling or resorting to excessive formality).

- *Demands to meet personal needs.* These may include insisting on talking about personal experiences to the detriment of participation by others, asking for help to draw attention to self, or special pleading in the form of introducing pet themes or claiming to speak for the 'grass roots'.

- *Excessive aggression and competition.* These may include criticizing or blaming others, interrupting, taking over the discussion, referring only to the group leader, denigrating the contributions of others or asserting authority.

Another type of problem may be *failure to participate*. Some group members may avoid contributing, perhaps because of shyness, low self-esteem, or self-perceived lack of communication skills. Occasionally a member may fail to participate because he or she is an unwilling or uninterested participant.

FIGURE 5.2   *A sociogram*

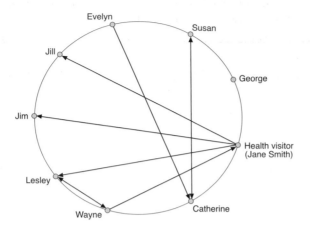

Representing a class of eight secondary school students who were discussing drug dependency in their city. The health visitor is acting as facilitator to the group discussion. The lines indicate the number of comments made in the 15 minutes the observer recorded. The arrows indicate the direction of the comments. For example, Jane Smith directed comments to Jim, Jill and Lesley. George was not involved at all. This analysis illustrates who spoke and to whom.

Every group member can play a part in reducing potential problems, but clearly the leader has a special responsibility for minimizing self-centred behaviour and drawing out reluctant members. Whatever the problem, it is important to be sensitive to the possible reasons underlying the behaviour, and to deal with them in a supportive rather than destructive manner.

Monitoring group process

Groups form best and learn or work most when they are encouraged to monitor process, or what is going on in the group. In situations where there is a clear intention to minimize the dependency on a professional health teacher, monitoring of group process is particularly important, and teaching group members to observe and record group process will be an essential part of the health teacher's role.

The role of the observer in a group is to monitor and record what is going on, to interpret what is seen and heard and to report it to the group. The observer has to be able to give an honest account, including pointing out any problems that may be developing. The observer role is not as straightforward as it may seem; observers have to consider verbal, nonverbal and extraverbal behaviour. It requires skill to interpret behaviour without judging the person. A group needs feedback on group building and maintenance, group progress towards accomplishing tasks, group style, and group interaction, including self-oriented behaviour.

Process recording techniques. A technique useful for inexperienced observers is the sociogram. It requires mapping out the positions of group members and then drawing arrows to indicate the direction of any verbal interaction. Figure 5.2 shows a sociogram drawn during the first few minutes of a discussion group looking at a drug problem. The person who records the sociogram should be asked to interpret it for the rest of the class and lead discussion on its interpreta-

BOX 5.2	*Example of an observer's brief*

- Your role as observer is to give feedback to the group about how they are tackling their health learning or health-related problem.
- Concentrate on what you see and hear people doing rather than what you think they may be feeling.
- You are to note the behaviour of group members, and comment on individual contributions to group maintenance or group task functions.
- You should also record examples of self-centred behaviour.

BOX 5.3	*Example of a recording sheet used to analyse group member participation*

Here is a list of behaviour observable in most groups:

Task functions	*Group building*	*Self-centred behaviour*
Initiating	Encouraging	Diverting the group
Information seeking	Compromising	Withdrawing
Information giving	Bringing others in	Interruption
Opinion giving	Setting standards	Denigrating others
Elaborating	Relieving tension	Rejecting ideas
Summarizing	Listening	Dominating discussion

Note below examples of any of the above that you see during the group's work.

Behaviour	*By (name)*	*To (name)*	*Reminder notes*

tion. Another technique is to ask one or two members to note evidence of group building and maintenance of group task functions being undertaken, or self-centred behaviour displayed. People learning to observe should be briefed about their role (see Box 5.2) and given a simple recording sheet to help them in their task (see Box 5.3). It may be possible to arrange for the group members to observe themselves in action by using video recording facilities.

As a teaching method, group work lends itself particularly well to learning within the affective domain. Attitudes, beliefs, values and opinions can be discussed, questioned and clarified. The small group session can also be an effective setting within which the learners' understanding of cognitive material can be explored, and questions can be addressed, in order to facilitate deep-level learning.

Demonstration

Nurses and midwives have numerous teaching opportunities that entail the teaching of psychomotor skills. Commonly such teaching sessions consist of a narrated demonstration by the health teacher, practice by the learner (patient

ACTIVITY 5.1

Think of a group you have participated in recently. This might be a seminar or discussion group in class, a staff meeting in a practice placement area, a student activity group, and so on. Describe the characteristics of the group:

- Who led the group, and who were the members?
- What was the group's purpose?
- What leadership style was used?
- How was the task of the group accomplished?
- Did problems arise with any of the members? If so, what types of problems were they? Were they resolved, and if so how? If they were not, how might they have been resolved?
- Did the group achieve its purpose? How might it have been more effective?

Keep these questions in mind, and repeat the exercise the next time you participate in a group.

or client), feedback on performance, and repeat demonstration, practice and feedback as necessary.

Teaching new mothers how to bath a baby provides a typical example of such a teaching opportunity. First the organization of materials is shown, then the undressing of the baby with discussion of safety concerns such as keeping a steadying hand on the baby to prevent falling. Later the bathing of the baby is done, demonstrating the 'top-to-bottom', 'clean-to-unclean' principles. Finally, the end of the demonstration includes drying and clothing the baby and also care of the umbilical cord area. Frequently, this kind of demonstration includes advice on nappy (diaper) rash, checking the fontanelle, and dry skin care. There is a great deal of useful information which can be given, and mothers may feel overwhelmed. A repeat demonstration in parts may be helpful: organization of bath materials, handling and undressing the baby, bathing, and after-care. Time for discussion and feedback is essential. The need for repetition of the demonstration, followed by practice with supervision, should be decided by both the mother and the nurse or midwife. The extent of learning may be assessed through repeated practice sessions.

Preparing a demonstration requires as much thought and prior preparation as any other form of teaching. It should not be assumed that the skilled performer will automatically demonstrate adequately. There are a number of things to plan for:

- *Clarify the purpose.* It is important to decide exactly what has to be demonstrated, and why. The demonstration should concentrate on the skill to be achieved; it is not appropriate to include all aspects of related learning.
- *Be sure the demonstration is seen.* A common reason for demonstrations not being seen is that they happen too quickly. The object of the exercise is for the individual to gain confidence that the skill will be mastered; a swift professional execution can often have exactly the opposite effect. It could be argued that a smooth performance at normal speed can be useful

in the first instance, to let the learners see what the eventual goal is, but this should be followed by a demonstration in which they have time to observe the elements of the procedure. The ideal speed for demonstration of injection technique, for instance, may be considerably slower than the usual speed of administration, with pauses between steps in the procedure.

Some things need to be seen in close-up, and this will either limit the size of the group or necessitate the use of audiovisual material, such as video or larger-than-life models. Use of video or computer-based projection has obvious benefits in providing close-ups. On the other hand, taking the object to be seen in close-up 'live' to group members singly or in pairs has the additional advantage that they can touch the materials and ask questions immediately. For close-ups, it is important to get the perspective right, and if possible it is best to avoid presenting a mirror image.

- *Limit distractions.* Only essential items should be included in the demonstration itself. In teaching tooth brushing, for instance, the range of toothbrushes and pastes should be displayed separately; likewise, in teaching stoma care, the range of appliances should be discussed before or after the technique of changing the bag is demonstrated. During the demonstration itself, discussing the full range of items which potentially could be relevant is distracting. Unnecessary or ill-timed commentary is also distracting, so this needs to be thought out ahead of time.

- *Organize the sequence.* A demonstration can be organized by showing the complete skilled performance initially and then examining component skills. Another possibility is to show individual difficult parts first, and then demonstrate the full skilled performance. For instance, there may be an advantage in alerting learners to a wrist position or how a syringe is filled so that they may look out for these aspects when watching complete injection technique. People learn differently and it is most important to be alert to signs that indicate understanding or lack of it.

- *Prepare for repetition.* Parts of the demonstration that deal with vital or difficult aspects should be repeated. The nurse knows which aspects are vital and can plan for these. Identifying other difficulties can be done on an individual basis with the learner.

- *Think through the details.* It is important to make provision for such items as electricity or water supply, waste disposal and protective clothing. For demonstrations to be clear and uninterrupted, all necessary items of equipment should be on hand and in working order.

- *Arrange follow-up.* The whole or parts of the demonstration may have to be repeated. Practice, initially with supervision, should be available to the learner soon after the demonstration.

- *Provide feedback.* Once the learner practises the skill, he or she needs to know what is being done correctly and what needs further refinement. Only in this way can improvement in the skill be achieved. In addition, feedback can enhance motivation, and it is important to remember to highlight the positive as well as any negative aspects of the learner's performance.

Demonstration is a technique that is well suited to the teaching of psychomotor skills, but it is also a good opportunity to integrate cognitive and affective aspects of learning. The health teacher can highlight the relationship between elements from the three domains as the demonstration and practice progress.

Role play

Role play can be used to demonstrate opinions and feelings and to identify coping skills. It is often described as an 'experiential' learning technique, because it enables participants to engage in experience, albeit pretend experience. This element of pretence allows the learner to experience near-realism without the risks that might be inherent in real-life experience.

Role playing makes use of drama technique, with learners acting assigned parts. Usually the playing out of roles is improvised. For instance, in learning how to use communication techniques, the parents of an adolescent with whom they have been having difficulty communicating can role play with the teacher, who can take the role of the adolescent. Subsequent analysis of the interaction is an essential part of role play.

To initiate a role play, the scene should first be set, then the actors' roles are defined. Roles may be assigned or volunteers requested, depending on the circumstances and purpose of the activity. Directions regarding the situation begin the role play. For instance, in the example given above, the teacher might say, 'I'll play the part of your adolescent son and we are discussing whether or not I can go out with my friends to a rave on a Saturday night'. Equally, it can be useful to ask one of the parents to play the part of the son, since this may help them to gain insight into their son's feelings and point of view.

After a short period of interaction, at a logical point, the role play should be stopped and analysis begun. Discussion of the interaction should come from all participants (including the audience if one is present) and learning may occur in several ways. In the instance of the parent–son role play:

- The parents may identify why their adolescent son doesn't talk with them, or grows silent in discussions about his behaviour.

- Suggestions about other ways to approach their son may be formulated when the identified communication patterns appear inadequate.

- The parents may wish to learn other communication techniques to try with their son.

- The parents may feel less frustrated and more willing to accept a changed level of communication (temporary or permanent) with their son.

Many difficult areas of communication and feelings can be addressed using role play: young people learning to negotiate personal and sexual relationships; communicating with a dying relative; interaction between a person in a wheelchair and an able-bodied person; and so on. Because such issues are often difficult and emotive, it is crucial that the participants in role play have the opportunity to de-brief or de-role once the interaction has taken place. This entails allowing the players to be themselves again, acting as themselves, and to express their feelings about the role play experience.

Role play can be particularly useful for learning in the affective domain as well as the psychomotor domain. However, it is also a good way to draw in a number of complex aspects of learning at the same time, potentially in all three domains and at various levels.

ACTIVITY 5.2

Read through ALL the directions for this activity before beginning.

Have you had an argument or serious difference of opinion with someone recently? Get together with a friend or classmate and outline the circumstances to him or her. Now ask your partner to role play you while you role play the other party in re-enacting your disagreement. It would be helpful to have a third person observe while you are doing this.

Once you and your fellow player have worked your way through the situation, discuss with each other your feelings about it. Did you learn anything about the other person's point of view? Did your partner gain an understanding of how you felt?

After your discussion, be sure you have both returned to being yourselves before you leave the role play setting.

Important note: For your psychological safety (and for the sake of your friendship with your role play partner!), do not select a situation that is too painful or risky, in emotional terms. And if either of you should begin to find things too difficult during the role play, STOP – or call 'time out'. This is meant to be a healthy exercise for you! Your observer, if you have one, can be helpful in this respect, by watching for danger signs.

CHOOSING TEACHING TECHNIQUES AND AIDS

Choice of technique

The choice of technique will be directed by the objectives the teacher and the learner wish to achieve. Other considerations in selection include the number of participants, the type of material to be learned and the kind of learning to be promoted. There is no exact way of determining which teaching techniques will work. Much depends on the personal styles of both learner and teacher.

The teaching methods discussed in this chapter do not constitute an exhaustive list of methods; there are others. They do represent a useful range, however. In general, methods can be divided into two types: those that are primarily didactic, that is, those that involve the transmission of information, and those that are experiential, that is, those that involve active experience for the learners. The lecture is the most didactic, while the most experiential could be said to be real life. Didactic methods are most successful for learning in the cognitive domain, though even then, if they are used alone they may not be able to achieve more than surface-level learning. Experiential methods can be the best means of achieving learning in the psychomotor and affective domains. Here again, though, experiential methods alone may not be sufficient; some didactic teaching may be necessary if the learning is to be informed. Ideally, experiential methods can provide a setting in which the relationship between knowledge and action (theory and practice) can be clarified.

Table 5.1 provides a quick reference to a variety of techniques, with indications of their use and a note of advantages and disadvantages.

TABLE 5.1	*Teaching techniques*

What the health teacher hopes to accomplish	Kind of learning	Technique	Learner activity status	Advantages	Disadvantages	Example
1. Present information for consideration	Cognitive	■ Lecture ■ Panel ■ Reading ■ Audiovisual aids e.g. films, video, computer programmes	Passive	■ Economical of time and resources ■ Can teach large number of learners ■ Learners feel secure in large group ■ Large amount of information can be presented	■ Does not promote interaction or problem-solving ■ Teacher cannot check individual progress ■ Same learning pace for all ■ Learner-attractiveness low	A group of mothers of babies with hydrocephalus learn about the condition and how the shunt mechanism works
2. Develop skills – interpersonal, psychomotor, etc.	Cognitive Psychomotor Affective	■ Demonstration and return demonstration ■ Simulation ■ Role play	Active	*For 2, 3 & 4* ■ Learner involvement ■ Permits interaction ■ Facilitates evaluation by teacher ■ Enables learner to risk in secure environment ■ Develops problem solving skills, self-evaluation ■ Provides closer approximation to reality ■ Allows more variation in pace to suit learner	*For 2, 3 & 4* ■ High cost in time and resources ■ Socialising may decrease concentration ■ Difficult to standardize learning for all learners ■ Shyness may inhibit some learners from participating ■ With computer-based learning a lonely way to learn, may encourage a rigid view of correct responses	A patient with a leg injury learns to use crutches
3. Encourage understanding	Cognitive Possibly affective	■ Problem-solving exercises ■ Group participation ■ Guided project work ■ Computer-based learning with feedback	Active			An adolescent with diabetes learns to understand and come to terms with her diabetes and relate to others with diabetes
4. Encourage examination of attitudes and values	Affective Cognitive	■ Group work, sharing experiences – counselling – games – role play – discussion – debate	Active			A young man learns about possible consequences of his drug-taking lifestyle

Choice of aid

Appropriate use of teaching aids can enrich the teaching and learning process. The stimulation of several senses helps to engage the learner more fully. It is beyond the scope of this text to deal in detail with the use of aids, but Table 5.2 provides a useful check list on a range of teaching aids which are available. There is an increasing variety of 'high-tech' aids on the market. Some of these, such as interactive CD-ROM, can be useful, though they may be less readily

TABLE 5.2   *Teaching aids Adapted from Hardy 1983*

Aid	Advantages	Disadvantages	Example
1. Printed matter – books, handouts	■ Allows self-pacing ■ Learners can refer back to it when required ■ Reduces need for note-taking and related anxiety ■ Handouts can be made specific to individual learning needs ■ Can supplement teaching session	■ Books are expensive and rapidly out-of-date ■ Handouts must be planned carefully and used appropriately, and cannot replace teaching ■ Copyright law limits mass duplication of material	In a discussion of nutrition, handouts about essential food groups and whether family members are eating a well-balanced diet
2. Models of life, e.g. skeleton	■ Three-dimensional ■ Resemble reality ■ Allow for close examination ■ Allow for practice ■ Stimulate visual and tactile senses	■ May be expensive ■ Useful for small groups only ■ Are not the same as reality	Use of a doll in antenatal class demonstrations for expectant parents
3. Real specimens, equipment	■ Present reality ■ Three-dimensional ■ Stimulate visual and tactile senses	■ May not be easily available ■ Useful for small groups only ■ May be expensive, difficult to store	Use of real baby in demonstrating baby bathing procedure
4. Graphics – charts, posters, drawings, photographs	■ Stimulate visual sense ■ Promote organization and correlation of material ■ Help to approximate reality ■ Easily stored and retrieved ■ May not require teacher presence	■ Production of materials needs to be of high standard ■ Useful for small groups only	Poster showing major elements of diabetic self-care, displayed in diabetic outpatient clinic
5. Blackboard, whiteboard, flipchart	■ Stimulate visual sense ■ Inexpensive ■ Can accommodate fairly large audience ■ Allows for development of presentation ■ Versatile, usable for various purposes	■ Skill needed for effective use ■ Danger of attending to board rather than audience during presentation ■ Material erased and no longer available for inspection or review (flipchart pages can be retained)	Use in a class with diabetics to illustrate the production and function of insulin in the body
6. Flannel board, magnetic board, bulletin board	■ Easy to assemble and use, may be portable ■ Can be used repeatedly ■ Teacher and learners can participate ■ Stimulates visual sense	■ Limited usefulness, depending on context and learning need	For a group of teenage mothers, selecting and arranging food items for a well-balanced daily diet

Continued overleaf

TABLE 5.2 cont	*Teaching aids* Adapted from Hardy 1983

Aid	*Advantages*	*Disadvantages*	*Example*
7. Field trips	■ Motivating and interesting ■ Active learner involvement ■ Presentation of reality	■ Costly of time in organizing and accomplishing ■ Requires transport ■ Appropriate for small groups only	For a group of people with learning disabilities, a visit to shops to assess appropriate selection of clothing items
8. Overhead projection	■ Stimulates visual sense ■ Relatively easy to prepare and use ■ Can be used with large audience ■ Can be either pre-planned or used on the spot ■ Can be used to illustrate process stages and develop material ■ Can allow for learner participation	■ Electricity supply needed ■ Equipment moderately costly ■ Transparencies must be planned carefully to be effective	For a group of patients with renal failure, to explain kidney function and how dialysis works to substitute for this
9. Photographic slides, film strips	■ Can be used with large audience ■ Can be adapted for use in self-directed learning programmes ■ Relatively easy reproduction ■ Stimulate visual and sometimes auditory senses	■ Need partial darkness for viewing ■ Careful planning of slide order of presentation is needed ■ User must be proficient with the equipment	For patients with recent colostomies, slide presentation of appliance management
10. 'Powerpoint' presentations	■ Can be used with projector for large audience or computer screen for individuals or small groups ■ Presentation can be easily tranported on computer, 'floppy disk' or CD, or sent electronically ■ May stimulate both visual and auditory senses ■ Can incorporate a variety of types of visual material, e.g. text, graphs, photos	■ Time and skill are needed for preparation ■ Depends on use of expensive equipment to project/display ■ Teacher needs to be competent with use of equipment ■ Inexpertly produced presentations can be boring	For a group of people with weight problems, information about activity and diet, with film clip incorporated of formerly obese people describing their experience of being obese and losing weight
11. Films, videos, television	■ Resemble reality ■ Can be used with large or small audiences ■ Can illuminate attitudes and values and demonstrate skills ■ Stimulate visual and auditory senses	■ Need careful selection and previewing ■ Need meaningful introduction and follow-up discussion ■ Equipment is costly ■ Electricity supply required ■ May include inappropriate or irrelevant material	With high school students, cases of drug dependency viewed and used as a basis for discussion

TABLE 5.2 cont	**Teaching aids** *Adapted from Hardy 1983*		

Aid	*Advantages*	*Disadvantages*	*Example*
12. Tape recordings	■ Stimulate auditory sense ■ Self-pacing is possible ■ Can be used with small or large audiences ■ Relatively inexpensive ■ Can be battery-operated	■ Good quality recordings may be difficult to obtain ■ User must be proficient with equipment	Initial session of a group discussing health attitudes is taped; at a later meeting the tape is played back and discussed
13. Expert contributors	■ Present reality ■ May provide a point of comparison ■ May command respect because of knowledge ■ Nature of 'expertise' can be widely varied – e.g. professionals, patients, politicians	■ May not be easily available ■ May be expensive ■ Teacher has only limited control over material presented	An adolescent diabetic who copes well with his condition speaks to a group of new juvenile diabetics about how he feels about his condition and its management

available to the health teacher, and they may not meet the individual needs of a particular learning situation.

Teaching aids have to serve the purposes of both learner and teacher, as well as fitting the resources available. A number of questions should be considered in choosing an aid:

- Will it add to interest or understanding, or is it merely a distraction, or a prop for the teacher?
- Will it be acceptable to the learner?
- Will it provide the opportunity for transfer of learning?
- Will it involve the learner?
- Is it appropriate to the learner's age, ability and experience?
- Is it flexible?
- Is it readily available?
- Is it worth the cost?
- Can the teacher use it with ease?
- What contribution will it make to achieving the objectives for learning?

Only if such questions engender positive answers should the aid be used. A poor or inappropriate aid can be detrimental rather than helpful to the teaching–learning process. A good aid, on the other hand, can be a valuable adjunct to the teacher's contribution; sometimes indeed 'a picture is worth a thousand words'.

ACTIVITY 5.3

Think of three health teaching topics, one primarily cognitive in content, one primarily psychomotor, and the other primarily affective. How easy do you find it to separate the topics into the three domains? For each of the topics you have chosen, identify who your learners would be. What is it you would want these people to learn? Consider the methods that would be most appropriate to achieve the learning that would be needed. Can you think of any audiovisual aids that would help to achieve the learning goal?

REFERENCES

Benne KD, Sheats P 1948 Functional roles and group members. Journal of Social Issues 4(2): 41-49.

Davis BG 1993 Tools for teaching. San Francisco, Jossey-Bass.

Dean B 2001 Zimbabwe's eager pupils are too poor to practise what they learn. The Guardian, Monday June 25, 2001.

Dean J, Kenworthy N 2000 The principles of learning. In: Nicklin P J, Kenworthy N (eds) Teaching and assessing in nursing practice: an experiential approach, pages 45-67. Edinburgh, Ballière Tindall.

Hardy LK 1983 Self-appraisal in health. Scottish Health Education Group, Edinburgh.

Lewin K 1947 Frontiers in group dynamics. Human Relations 1: 5-42.

Ley P 1976 Towards better doctor patient communications: contributions from social and experimental psychology. In: Bennett A E (ed) Communication between doctors and patients. Nuffield Provincial Hospitals Trust, Oxford University Press, Oxford.

Ley P, Spelman MS 1965 Communications in an out-patient setting. British Journal of Social and Clinical Psychology 4: 114-116.

Meade CD 1988 Effect of document simplification on patients' comprehension. Unpublished PhD thesis, University of Illinois at Chicago.

Pratt L, Seligman A, Reader G 1957 Physicians' views on the level of medical information among patients. The American Journal of Public Health 47: 1277.

SPW 2003 HSPW Zimbabwe health education programmes. Students Partnership Worldwide, London http://www.spw.org/zimbabwe/healtheducationprogrammes.htm Accessed April 14, 2003.

Thorne SE, Hislop G, Harris S, Nelems B 2002 Toward effective patient-professional communication in cancer care, 2001-2004. Research proposal, National Cancer Institute of Canada. http://www.bccrc.ca/ccr/ghislop_project4.html Accessed August 8, 2003.

White R, Lippett R 1968 Leader behaviour and member reaction in three social climates. In: Cartwright D, Zander A (eds) Group dynamics: research and theory, 3rd edn. Tavistock Publications, London.

2 THE PROCESS OF HEALTH TEACHING

6 Beginning the teaching–learning process: assessment of learning needs

This chapter addresses the first stage in the teaching learning process. In common with many versions of the problem-solving process, including the nursing process, the teaching learning process begins with assessment. This is often referred to more specifically as a needs assessment.

ASSESSMENT AND THE CONCEPT OF NEED

The purpose of the needs assessment is to identify the client's needs for learning with respect to his or her health. Achieving this entails the identification of what the client needs to know, what his or her present state of knowledge is, and determining the difference between the two. The difference, or *learning deficit*, thus calculated constitutes the client's *learning needs*. Throughout this chapter it is assumed that the identification of deficits is an integral part of defining needs.

Professionals and patients may differ in their interpretation of what needs to be learned and why, so assessment has the best chance of success when the teacher and learner work together. Of course, there may have to be exceptions to this, such as when someone is too ill to take part or is unwilling or unable to accept responsibility. There are three aspects of the assessment process: collection of information, analysis of information and identification of learning needs (see Figure 6.1).

The three steps of assessment are interrelated and are not necessarily sequential, in the strict sense. Neither nurses nor clients begin the assessment process with a mental 'blank sheet of paper'. Each nurse has a mental framework based on experience of previous patients with similar needs. Clients have

FIGURE 6.1   *Assessment: systematic, continuous, productive*

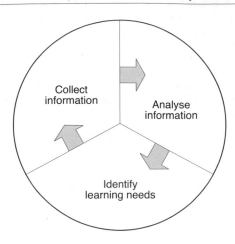

ideas about themselves and their own lives, and may also have preconceptions of what is likely to be involved in certain illnesses and what may be expected of them. The type of analysis the data will be subjected to influences information-gathering for assessment, and this depends on assumptions about the kind of teaching objectives which are likely to be set.

A fundamental issue in assessment revolves around the concept of 'need'. Some definitions or statements about nursing discuss 'need' as if it were an absolute. This is not the case; on the contrary, it is a relative term. Not only are needs perceived differently by different people, but they also change over time.

Chambers and his colleagues (1980) identified that the words 'want', 'need', 'demand', 'use' and 'supply' may all refer to the same thing or may reflect different conceptual approaches depending on the orientation of the individuals considering them. Categorizing needs helps to clarify what is meant and to alert the health teacher to differing views. Bradshaw (1972) described a taxonomy of needs that has been widely used around the world and across a range of disciplines. His taxonomy included four types of needs:

■ *Normative needs.* These are defined by health care experts based on their assessment of the client's status in relation to an accepted standard (the 'norm'). They are neither absolute nor objective; instead, they reflect professional judgements. Value judgements may also play a role as professionals have value sets of their own. For these reasons even the experts may disagree about aspects of need. Definitions of normative needs may conflict with the client's view of his own needs.

■ *Felt needs.* These needs are those perceived by the client. Demand for given services may be limited by the perceptions of individuals. In order to feel the need for a service, the health consumer has to be aware that it may be available. A person may feel a need without being able to articulate it, thus the need may or may not be expressed.

■ *Expressed needs.* These arise from felt needs, but are demonstrated in words or action. The client asks questions, joins or forms a self-help group, or demands a service, all of which actions express a need. Health teachers' assessments cannot rely only on expressed needs, because clients are not always aware of their needs, and even when they are, they may not ask or act to try to meet them.

■ *Comparative needs*. By studying similar populations it is possible to identify expressed needs and services which exist in one population but not in another. The observed difference may prompt the conclusion that such need exists in the population under study. Frequently, though not always, this is a matter of expert opinion. In addition, the presence or lack of service may not relate to need, depending on the reasons for introducing the service in the first place.

The difficulties associated with the definition of 'need' highlight the importance of client participation in assessment. In this respect, a particularly useful aspect of Bradshaw's taxonomy is that it prompts the user to look at needs from a range of perspectives, not just from the professional point of view.

Individuals will express some needs freely and articulately. Other needs are not so readily verbalized. Many people find it difficult to say what they want and need to know about their health. Possible reasons may include, for example, lack of familiarity with technical terms, embarrassment, feelings of social distance from health care professionals, denial of illness, pain, lack of privacy, or a belief that expressing the need would be futile. It is a common experience to be vague or to have mixed feelings about health-related information. Thus felt needs often exceed expressed needs.

An important part of the collection of information for learning assessment is therefore concerned with ascertaining how nearly the expressed needs of a client reflect the felt needs. In assessing client-perceived needs, the nurse has to be ready to take into account what the individual has to say. It may also be necessary to note what is not said, or to determine whether what is said is what is meant. Clearly, the processes of data gathering and data analysis are interdependent.

Perception of need: the client's view

Research has found that, when asked about care, recently discharged hospital patients frequently criticize the lack of information (Cartwright 1964; Hugh-Jones et al 1964; Raphael 1977). Poor explanations have also proved dissatisfying to patients (Skipper et al 1964), while medical language has acted as a barrier to understanding (Linehan 1966; Reynolds 1978). In a study of patients undergoing day surgery, Mitchell (2000) investigated differences between 'vigilant copers' (those who wanted maximum information) and 'avoidant copers' (those who wanted minimal information) and found that when patients were mismatched with the amount of information provided, the vigilant copers who received too little information were the most anxious. A study by Pearson (2001) found that patients who had undergone emergency surgery indicated that adequate information was one of the essential factors that enabled them to regain control of their lives.

Fear of pain and fear of the unknown are frequently described as concerns that imply needs. Reynolds (1978) found that people feared the unknown more than they feared the truth. Koivula et al (2002) carried out a study looking at the relationship of social support to fear and anxiety in patients awaiting coronary artery bypass grafts. One of their findings was that patients with high fear levels perceived a greater need for information than did patients with lower fear levels.

Most people therefore want information, but a few may not. Cartwright (1964) reported that 33% of a sample of 739 ex-hospital patients wanted to know 'as much as possible' about their diseases, but 10% of the same sample were consistently passive, not wanting much information nor asking questions. Benson et al (1977) found that patients wanted comprehensive information about intrauterine devices. In contrast, McIntosh (1976) discovered that the majority of subjects did not want to know more and described a situation in which lack of insight gave people hope. Such conflicting results reinforce the necessity for individual assessment.

Differences in desire for type as well as amount of information should be expected. Eardley et al (1975) found that people varied in the amount and type of advice they wanted. Needs have been found to vary with social class (Beal & Dickson 1974; Samson et al 1971; Henshaw 2001) and intelligence (Sims 1977). Dodge (1969) described patients' information-seeking as 'survivalist'. The patients in her study attended to information they thought was important. In rank order, the items were: diagnosis, results of tests, aetiology of condition, future long-term effects and temporary activity restrictions. A number of other studies have confirmed that diagnosis is of primary concern to the individual patient (see reviews by Ley & Spelman 1967; Hayward 1975). Okun and Rice (2001) found that when elderly patients with osteoarthritis were provided with teaching material about their disease, their recall was more accurate for information that confirmed what they already believed than for information that disagreed with their prior beliefs.

Perception of need: the nurse's view

Do nurses' perceptions of need differ from those of clients? Earlier it was suggested that they do. An example of this may be a case where the nurse assumes that the client needs to know why his diet is restricted while he, on the other hand, may be interested only in what the restrictions are and how long they will be imposed. Equally, it could arise that the nurse assumes the patient requires to know only that premedication before surgery will cause drowsiness, while the patient feels entitled to know what the medication is called and how quickly it will take effect. Obviously, such differences in perception are unhelpful. They can and should be cleared up by a few minutes of discussion.

On the other hand, some differences in perception of need may assist the process of assessment. The nurse has experience with other patients and knowledge of research to draw on in identifying needs. This can be used to help patients identify or verbalize their needs.

Research has revealed something of how patients' and nurses' perceptions of need differ. Dodge (1972) found that patients valued information about long-term effects, how they would feel, how the illness was going to affect them, the degree of disability they would suffer, how lifestyles would be altered, their progress, diagnosis and prognosis, what was expected of them and how well they were coping with the condition. Contrary to these expectations were the nurses' perceptions of need, which included information on hospital routine and policy, timing of events, geography of the ward and relevant parts of the hospital, who's who on the staff, knowledge of investigations and treatment, what to expect during and after treatment, how they would feel after treatment, and precautions and limitations associated with treatment. Different perceptions of need have been recorded by other investigators (Pratt et al 1957; Ashworth 1978; Greene et al 1980). Such findings have obvious implications for the most basic teaching that takes place when a patient is admitted to hospital or first learns of an illness problem.

Barriers to the perception of needs

While it is essential for the health teacher to take account of the patient's or client's view of his or her needs if learning is to be successful, there are times when the teacher may be aware of a need when the client is not. Then the impetus for the teaching–learning activity will need to come from the professional. An example of this can be seen in a study of 'wet work employees' by Held et al (2002). Such employees might not be aware of the danger of developing skin problems, but the occupational health professional will be well aware of such dangers. A study by Katz et al (2002) found that only 36% of parents of children with sickle cell disease realised that their affected children were at risk of suffering stroke as a complication. These parents would not be aware that they needed to know about the signs of stroke, and what to do if they developed, so it is up to the professional to identify the learning need. In such cases, although it may be the professional who identifies the need, it remains important that the measures taken to meet the need are tailored to the individual situation. As Ryan and Lauver (2002) found in an integrated review of the literature, tailored informational interventions have been shown to be more effective than standard interventions, and they are preferred by patients.

Even when patients or clients are aware of a need for information, they may be reluctant to express their need, as Linehan (1966) reported. Eardley et al (1975) found that morale and busyness of the ward affected patients' information-seeking.

Nurses may not always respond well to clients' attempts at expressing their needs. Faulkner (1980, 1981) explored nurses' conversation with patients and found that it was stereotyped and superficial and that they spent little time actually talking with patients. When student nurses were asked specific questions by patients, they had difficulty in providing answers and seemed to have no clear idea of their role in giving information to patients. Melia (1981, 1987) referred to the student-nurse experience as 'nursing in the dark', as the students she interviewed told her that the ward staff did not give adequate information regarding the patient. Kiger (1992, 1993, 1994) also found that student nurses felt a lack of information about patients, and a lack of agreement in amount or type of information given to them and given to the patients they were caring for. Such deficiencies and disparities make it virtually impossible for the qualified or student professional to carry out an adequate assessment of patients' learning needs.

Pohl (1965) and Redman (1971) suggested a range of factors which interfere with nurses taking full responsibility for patient teaching: lack of information, inadequate preparation, belief that sharing knowledge with patients will decrease nursing power, lack of time, inadequate staffing, lack of nursing service support, poor communication between members of the health care team, lack of information-seeking by patients and perceived reluctance of doctors to

| Box 6.1 | *Barriers to identification of needs* |

Teacher

Barriers to perception of client's needs:

- does not listen or respond to client's questions
- has insufficient information about client
- lacks knowledge to deal with questions
- discourages client participation to maintain control
- lacks time due to poor ward organisation, or inadequate staffing
- experiences little support from fellow professionals
- lacks confidence
- professional preparation has encouraged conservative beliefs about nurse's role in health teaching.

Learner

Barriers to expression of needs:

- reluctant to ask questions
- perceives ward too busy to seek attention
- lacks language to request technical information
- perceives professionals only as helpers, not teachers or informants
- adopts passive role readily
- not ready or motivated to participate
- convinced by previous experiences that expression of needs is not welcomed
- does not consider health teaching part of the nurse's role.

allow nurses to teach. Evidence existed (Marsh 1979; Carter 1981; Webster 1981) that nurses lacked relevant knowledge of teaching and had insufficient opportunity to practise teaching skills. Smith (1979) commented that a lack of commitment to health education may have played a significant role. Significant changes have taken place in nursing and midwifery education in many countries during the 1990s and the early 21st century, and these should bring about improvement in this situation. Health promotion now has a prominent place in pre-registration programmes in the UK, and principles of teaching and assessment have a high profile in both pre- and post-registration programmes.

Nurses may still need to change people's expectations of nurses as teachers if they are to help them articulate information needs. Cartwright (1964) found that 46% of patients expected doctors to be the main source of information while only 28% saw the ward sister as providing information. Nearly four decades later, Chelf et al (2002), in a study of patients with cancer attending an outpatient care setting, found that 64% of patients identified discussion with doctors as their most preferred means of learning about cancer topics. Only 34% identified discussion with nurses as another preferred means, with brochures or booklets rating nearly as highly at 33%.

Some barriers to accurate identification of needs are listed in Box 6.1.

The nurse's role as advocate in respect of need

In health care, needs appear to be limitless. In the UK, the proportion of the Gross Domestic Product (GDP) spent on the NHS has increased in every decade since its inception. In 1949, it was 3.9% of the GDP, in 1988 it was 5.8% (Office of Health Economics 1989), and in 1998 it was 6.8% (OECD 2001; Emmerson et al 2002). It is less than the average level of funding among EU countries, which in 1998 was 7.9% (OECD 2001; Emmerson et al 2002). In the USA, health care spending increased from 6.3% of Gross National Product (GNP) in 1967 to 13.6% in 1994 (Young & Bekeris 1999).

Despite this continuing increase in spending, unmet needs continue to exist. With recent economic recessions, and in the absence of a commitment to any significant increase in the proportion of investment in health care relative to other expenditure, health care systems in the western world are having to ration resources available for health care more than ever. This is done in a variety of ways: by allowing waiting lists to grow, either overtly or covertly; by increasing direct costs to the consumer; by limiting access by geographical region, age or clinical status, and so on. Examples of how such strategies can be operationalized might include: lengthening the procedure for getting on a waiting list; increasing prescription charges, or charging for dental and eye check-ups; concentrating a growing range of services in centres within major cities, making them less accessible to clients in rural areas; classifying all persons over a certain age as 'elderly' for all purposes, including urgent medical or surgical need; or withholding certain treatments from learning-disabled persons.

The nurse's role in assessing needs is crucial and can be seen to encompass two aspects: firstly, she must assess, comprehensively, the needs of individuals in her care, always conscious that their concept of need may differ from her own; and secondly, she must be capable of defining health education needs in general, in order to be able to make a case for resource allocation. At a time of economic stringency, with the government placing much emphasis on 'value for money', nurses have a particularly important part to play. In a general sense, nurses need to advocate the value of health education/promotion as a commodity. In an individual sense, the nurse needs to act as consumer advocate, establishing the case for the individual client's right to have adequate professionally-provided health teaching.

COLLECTING INFORMATION

The main source of relevant data on current learning needs is the person who is to be taught. Secondary sources of information include the family, friends and significant others, the client's doctors, previous health records, social records, developmental records such as those kept by health visitors and family general practitioners, and results of X-rays, laboratory tests and other investigations.

The simplest way to find out what someone needs to know is to ask him. Observation of his behaviour may also provide information. Asking the patient about his health learning needs can be surprisingly easy. Sometimes it

BOX 6.2	Areas for information seeking

Patient's/client's questions and comments

Anticipated needs (research based)

Diagnosis

Treatment

Investigations

Prognosis

Progress

Self-care

Routine

Aids/barriers to learning

Age

Cognitive state

Educational level

Emotional level

Grasp of technical language

Hearing

Comfort

Previous experience

Sex

Motivation to learn

Attitude

Learning ability

is enough just to arrange some privacy, set aside time, indicate interest and be prepared to listen. Often the first gathering of data on health teaching needs will happen when the patient is interviewed as part of the overall assessment of nursing needs. Felt needs are more likely to be expressed if the patient feels at liberty to ask questions. The secret of success in the nursing assessment interview may lie in conveying to the patient or client that questions will be welcomed and answered, if not by the interviewer, then by another health care professional. It may also be helpful to indicate that other opportunities to ask

ACTIVITY 6.1

Select a volunteer 'learner' from among your family and friends. With that person's permission, do an assessment of his or her health learning needs. In this case, your main source of information will be the individual him- or herself, as you will not have other professionals or health records to consult, but you will also have your own 'professional knowledge', values and views. For example, you can use your knowledge of Maslow's hierarchy to inform your assessment. (See Figure 6.3. on page 147)

What difficulties did you encounter in carrying out this activity? To what extent did your view and the person's own view of his or her health learning needs coincide? What does your analysis of the person's learning needs tell you about his or her teaching needs? How would you prioritise the learning/teaching needs you have identified?

Keep your notes on this activity for use during activities in later chapters.

questions are likely to occur and to suggest that the patient should jot down any questions which arise meantime.

What information should be sought? Complex forms for collecting data have been devised, but there are arguments about whether such forms are useful, or whether they tend to prejudge or circumscribe the relevant issues. As in any data-gathering session, general information must be recorded about the date of interview, the person's name, address, age, sex, religion, educational level and marital status. Box 6.2 illustrates three areas in which further information might be obtained. At an early point in the interview, the client's questions and comments should be elicited. This will give insight into the client's own perception of his or her needs and, as it introduces the session from the client's point of view, it may encourage continuing participation.

The way the person views his or her health situation should also be an area for assessment. For example, the questions below may help to discern the client's model of health:

- When have you been ill, and what caused your illnesses?
- Could you have prevented any of the illnesses you've had?
- What do you do that helps you to feel well?
- What do you do that makes you feel unwell?
- Do you feel you are as healthy as you can be?

In some settings it may be appropriate for the nurse to perform a physical assessment to complement the data reported in the health history and to provide objective evidence of the person's health status. This may provide one of the measures against which to evaluate the progress that results following health teaching. The nurse employs senses of sight, hearing, touch and smell through the four techniques of inspection, palpation, percussion and auscultation (see Box 6.3 for definitions).

Recording the results of the health history and physical examination is important for carrying out analysis of health learning needs and for communicating to other members of the health team. Recording expressed needs requires skill. It may be important, especially in an initial conversation, not to write down everything as it is said. Whenever possible it is advisable to give

BOX 6.3	*The four techniques of physical assessment*
Inspection:	to observe objectively and systematically, noting colour, odour and measurement as necessary.
Palpation:	to feel superficial and underlying structures of the body to note abnormalities.
Percussion:	to strike the surface of a body area with the fingers to produce sounds that will indicate the character of underlying tissue.
Auscultation:	to listen to sounds produced by the heart, lungs, blood vessels, abdominal organs.

full attention to what the patient is saying and to make arrangements for recording as soon afterwards as is feasible. Listing the patient's questions may be particularly useful. The number and type of questions may give clues as to the kind of information the patient wants and needs.

ANALYSING INFORMATION

Once initial information has been gathered, the analysis can begin. The purpose of analysis is to answer such questions as:

- How willing and able to learn is this person?
- How much does he or she need to know?
- What is the nature of the learning task?

Answers to these questions may be provided by using and building on information gathered in the initial assessment. Many experienced nurses can quickly detail what a patient needs to know in given circumstances. The more experienced they are, the more likely it is that they will also accurately determine how much the patient wants to know and is able to learn. Indeed, experienced nurses often collect and analyse information simultaneously, so in practice, the process by which such expert judgements are made is seldom recorded. Consequently, there is little direct evidence to instruct practice at this time.

At its simplest, however, the analysis must deal with balancing four areas of concern. These are: the present state of the patient's knowledge; what the patient says he or she needs to know about; what the nurse believes the patient needs to know about; and factors which are likely to affect the patient's ability and willingness to learn.

The current state of a person's knowledge, and his or her willingness and ability to learn, are affected by a number of factors. Age or developmental level, sex, education level and experience, language and level of anxiety were discussed in Chapter 3. Knowledge of such factors helps the nurse anticipate some general areas of concern. Clearly, the nurse may make some reasonably safe general assumptions about the different needs of a teenage female and an elderly man with the same diagnosis. What any particular person may need is a matter for more detailed consideration, however.

An obvious starting point for detailed individual analysis is with the list of questions asked by the patient at the initial assessment interview. Here again, the nurse must exercise judgement. Some questions clearly reveal considerable knowledge of diagnosis and a desire to get down to details. Others reveal ignorance or misinformation. But many questions cannot be interpreted at face value: pain, anxiety, first impressions of the health service, expectations and existing knowledge all affect what the individual may ask. Initial questions record what the person has been able to ask, and do not necessarily reflect all of what he wants and needs to know.

Going back to the patient's original questions provides the nurse with a platform for a second and more analytical interview. It also serves to demonstrate to the patient that his or her questions matter to the nurse and that the nurse is prepared to give the patient time to formulate further questions and seek the answers he or she wants.

The anticipated needs list prepared after the initial interview should also provide a framework for this second stage of assessment. The nurse will ask questions to ascertain how much the patient already knows about areas of importance that have been identified. Often this can be done by general discussion of the areas concerned. In complex situations, a check list or questionnaire may be useful.

Along with the assessment of learning needs and readiness to learn, it is necessary to consider the resources available for teaching. A main resource to consider is the nurse.

Yura and Walsh (1988) documented the knowledge framework nurses need in order to assess patients' health needs as including knowledge of communication and helping relationships, human anatomy and physiology, chemistry, physics, microbiology, psychology, sociology, cultural anthropology, comparative religions, developmental psychology, mathematics, literature, art, philosophy, theology, psychopathology and pathophysiology. In addition, the nurse as health teacher needs an up-to-date knowledge of relevant health statistics, with particular reference to subgroups in the population. The nurse also needs to have a knowledge of self and be aware of how his or her value judgements, prejudices and previous experience of illness and of health teaching may influence the resources he or she brings to bear on any particular teaching session. For instance, repeated failure with a particular type of client – the alcoholic, the obese person, the addicted cigarette smoker – may lead to undue pessimism; religious beliefs may make it difficult for the nurse to present options without bias in abortion counselling; unexplored feelings may block areas of discussion in counselling a bereaved person.

Clearly, the requisites detailed in the paragraph above constitute a tall order. They describe the ideal, perhaps a 'supernurse'. In reality, a critically important piece of self-knowledge for the nurse is an understanding of his or her own limitations, and this should be accompanied by a willingness to seek help as needed.

Another valuable resource in health teaching, but one that may be limited, particularly in clinical settings, is time. In the analysis of teaching needs, it is wise to consider realistically the time and personnel available for teaching. A teaching programme should be as comprehensive as possible, but there is no point in aiming at an all-embracing programme if it cannot be accomplished – that would be a recipe for failure.

Analysing the nature of the learning task

It is important to remember that most people who have something to learn about their health have an existing set of knowledge, beliefs and experience upon which to build. Often such background can be drawn on as a positive base for learning. Sometimes, however, the learning task may necessitate unlearning or relearning. How the person enters the teaching–learning situation may be coloured by vicarious as well as actual experience; that is, he or she may have learned from others' stories of their illness experiences or their contact with health care professionals. The person's attitudes towards these professionals should be elicited, because they may enhance or inhibit learning. A negative previous encounter may make a person reluctant to listen to information offered by nurses. In such an instance it will clearly take time to establish a position of trust.

Sometimes the unlearning of roles may have to occur before other more specific learning needs can be focused on. An example of this would be a woman who has had ulcerative colitis for years and in previous hospital experiences has tended to be a passive recipient of care. If she has an exacerbation of the condition that results in the need for an ileostomy, self-care will become an important teaching goal. Since she is accustomed to the nurse doing all the care, she may have to learn a new role as an active participant.

Analysis of the learning task also involves considering the types of learning required and the challenges they present to the individual learner. In reality, of course, the aspects of learning are interrelated. Nonetheless, some knowledge of the relative importance of each aspect may be helpful in selecting teaching methods, so an attempt should be made to consider the relative weight of aspects of learning. For instance, is the learning mainly cognitive, or are there important affective elements which may dictate the time and setting required for learning?

It can be difficult to weight the separate aspects of learning. What seem reasonable assumptions in general terms may have little validity in particular instances. For example, it may seem reasonable to assume that the nature of the disease or disability will dictate which aspects of learning are given precedence. Thus, cancer education may appear to be greatly concerned with emotional reactions and therefore affective learning. The individual cancer patient, however, may have already come to terms with the disease, perhaps through family experience, and may want to concentrate on acquiring information about the particular effects of current treatment. In the same vein, it might be assumed that people being prepared for surgery will require a cognitively based education programme, because of their obvious need for information, but an individual surgical patient may be frightened of surgery, and this could constitute a barrier to learning.

Such examples illustrate the relative merits and limitations of the assumption that the nature of the disease or condition determines the nature of the learning task. Clearly, the characteristics of the individual are at least as important as the nature of his or her illness. Relative weighting of factors is not as important as distinguishing the separate aspects of learning with respect to the challenges they pose to the individual.

A system of classifying types of learning in relation to teaching functions has been proposed (Bloom 1956; Krathwohl et al 1964). This suggests that there are levels of learning, and that they may be organized in a hierarchy of sophistication (see Chapter 3, Figure 3.3). In some situations health teaching may be minimal, because the learning is simple. The preoperative patient who has to fast for a period of time, for instance, needs only to have the information and understand the rationale for it. The person with a stoma, on the other hand, has to be able to apply new knowledge and understanding in caring for his stoma and to see relationships between stoma management and his lifestyle. In this case, the required learning is more complex.

Thus, in assessing the individual learner, certain questions can be posed:

- What type of learning is required, and at what level?
- Is the required cognitive learning concrete or abstract?
- Are the needed motor skills beyond the manual dexterity of the patient at 7 years or 70?
- Can the necessary affective learning be accomplished in the short term, or should interim goals be set?

Adults may have a clear idea of how they learn, so it may be possible to have the individual specify desired learning methods. It may also be helpful to ask the person how he usually learns things. What does he do when he has a number of things to remember? How did he go about learning his hobby? With children, it may be necessary to involve parents in discussion about how learning may be accomplished. There can never be a fixed formula, whether simple or complex, for predictable success in this area of assessment. Again, perhaps, the nature of the patient's questions and comments may give the best clues to this aspect of the educational task.

FIGURE 6.2   *Factors involved in analysis*

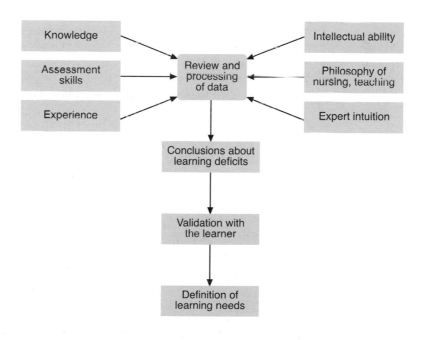

In analysis, all available information about the person, from subjective and objective sources, is reviewed and processed. Knowledge, skills, experience and sometimes expert intuition are used to interpret the data, and conclusions are drawn about the person's actual or potential learning needs. These are then validated with the patient or client (see Figure 6.2).

DEFINING LEARNING NEEDS

The assessment phase ends with the definition of the learning needs. In essence, the learning need is the statement which derives from the collection and interpretation of the data base and it is stated in a form which illustrates that an analytic approach helped to define it. For instance, a learning need might be stated:

> Mrs Smith needs to learn about stages of labour because she is seven months pregnant and is unable to describe or anticipate what she will experience when she begins her labour.

Listing learning needs helps to communicate to others the requirements for health teaching. The statements should be clear, simple, specific, concise and relevant to the nurse's role as health teacher. Occasionally the learning needs identified are beyond the scope of the nurse and should be referred to another health professional.

The list of learning needs implies a rank order of some kind. Usually, some needs require attention sooner than others. In the case of a newly diagnosed severe diabetic, learning about insulin and its effects would be a first priority, while diet could come later since the client's meals are prepared in hospital. Before going home, however, knowledge of nutrition would become a critical need.

Redman (1975) devised a system of prioritizing that is directly related to patient needs but also assumes professional experience and judgement. She has described three categories: acute educational needs, when lack of understanding is causing physical danger or psychosocial anguish; preventive educational needs, which exist when individuals are threatened by conditions they lack the skills to handle; and maintenance educational needs, which refer to needs of people who have to follow a medically prescribed regimen and may need frequent reteaching to maintain adequate levels of understanding and skill.

Maslow's hierarchy of needs may also provide a guide to assessing priorities. Maslow (1954) depicted human needs as falling into five categories. Starting with the most simple, on the lowest level of the hierarchy, *physiological needs* are basic to existence and include air, water, food, clothing and shelter. *Safety needs* relate to the need for survival. *Social or affiliative needs* (sometimes referred to as needs for 'love and belonging') are those which incorporate significant relationships. *Esteem needs* refer to those which enhance self-concept through achievement. Finally, *self-actualization needs*, at the highest level, involve the desire to achieve one's full potential in life (see Figure 6.3). When lower level needs are met, then needs at a higher level become prominent and require attention. There are, of course, exceptions and

FIGURE 6.3 *Maslow's hierarchy in simple form*

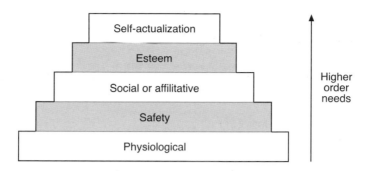

degrees of need. A person might be feeling hungry, yet a great interest in a subject being studied might keep the person's attention. Thus an absolute formula cannot be derived from Maslow's hierarchy, but it provides a useful guide to planning.

Use of Maslow's hierarchy of needs may be demonstrated in the case of the woman who has just been delivered of a normal healthy baby girl. Together, mother and midwife might list the learning needs and prioritize them thus:

Learning need and rationale	*Priority*
Self-care and recognition of normal postpartum physiological changes because she is going home in 48 hours and will need to do self-assessment	1
Baby care to ensure survival and development of child	1
Contraception because this pregnancy was unplanned	2
Parenting skills because she and her partner are first-time parents and have not attended parent-craft classes previously	2

Obviously the first two learning needs are immediately important for the survival of the mother and baby. The last two are important but can wait. Learning needs may thus be categorized as being short-term or long-term. Figure 6.4 summarizes the steps in assessment.

FIGURE 6.4   *The assessment process*

ASSESSMENT—with the client

- Collect information
  - from the learner about his or her health history
    and physical assessment, and from other sources,
    such as the family, the health record, etc
  - about the health teacher whose level of learning
    facilitation depends on his or her knowledge, ability
    and attitude

- Analyse the information
  - decide how willing and able the learner is
  - consider the nature of the learning tasks
    and decide on the challenges they present
    to teacher and learner

- Define the learning needs
  - refer to other teachers as necessary
  - prioritize

→ PLANNING

LEARNING NEEDS OF HEALTHY INDIVIDUALS AND GROUPS

In the discussion above, most of the examples given have been of individuals with an illness or injury, the major exception being examples related to child-birth. It should be remembered that healthy people also have health learning needs. As was pointed out in Chapter 1, *primary prevention* relates to the prevention of disease or disability before it occurs. Obviously such activity is often carried out with healthy people, though prevention of other disease and disability can, of course, be important for people who already have one disease problem.

Health teaching related to primary prevention is becoming more and more important, as the focus of health care moves increasingly away from the acute care setting and into the community. The nurse needs to be able to assess the needs of healthy people in order to plan preventive health teaching.

It is also important to remember that not all health teaching will be done with individuals. As was discussed in Chapter 5, there are times when teaching is planned for groups. Thus the health teacher needs to know how to assess the learning needs of groups, whether they are groups of people with health problems in common, or groups of healthy people.

Assessing the health learning needs of a group presents a particular challenge. The nurse may have no personal knowledge of any of the individuals in the group, yet if the teaching is to be successful, those individuals' needs must be taken into consideration. Although it may not be possible for the nurse to meet or know the individuals beforehand, it is still possible to obtain a certain

ACTIVITY 6.2

Imagine that you, as a nurse, have been asked to do a teaching session with a group of school children. They are in their sixth year of primary education and are a mixed group, about half girls and half boys, 25 children in all. The school is in a 'respectable' working-class neighbourhood. You have been told that you will have 50 minutes with them, and that you can select any health topic you think would be appropriate.

How will you decide what their health learning needs are? What information will you need, and where will you seek it? Suggest several topics you think might be appropriate, then prioritize them and select one that you would address in your teaching session. Why did you select that one? Having settled on a topic, how would you define the teaching needs, with respect to the session you would plan?

Keep your notes on this activity for use in an activity in a later chapter.

amount of information about them as a group, and to make a few 'educated guesses' about their characteristics. For example, a nurse who is asked to speak to a women's group about the menopause can find out how many women will be attending and what their age range is. She may be able to estimate their social class and likely educational level by the type and location of the group. All these factors will have implications for the style of presentation, the language used, the way to frame the topic, and so on. For instance, the perspective taken on the topic would need to be different for a group of middle-aged women going through, or on the verge of going through, the menopause, and for a group of young women for whom the menopause currently had more to do with their mothers than themselves.

It is helpful when teaching a group to allow time for questions and discussion, rather than trying to fill the allocated time with presentation. This can enable the health teacher to be more personal in assessing the needs of the individual participants, and the group as a whole. What questions are asked? What is the level of understanding shown? What misunderstandings are evident? What particular areas of interest are indicated? Thus some of the needs assessment can be done while the teaching is being carried out.

Assessment of needs, and the identification and prioritizing of the learning tasks, are useful in providing the basis for evaluating the success of health learning, and thus health teaching. This area is addressed later in this book.

REFERENCES

Ashworth AP 1978 Communication in the intensive care unit. Nursing Mirror 146(7): 34-36.

Beal JF, Dickson S 1974 Social differences in dental attitude and behaviour in West Midland mothers. Public Health 89(1): 19-30.

Benson H, Gordon L, Mitchell C 1977 Patient education and intrauterine contraception: a study of two package inserts. American Journal of Public Health 67(5): 446-449.

Bloom BS (ed) 1956 Taxonomy of educational objectives, handbook I: cognitive domain. David McKay, New York.

Bradshaw J 1972 A taxonomy of social needs. In: McLachlan G (ed) Problems and progress in medical care. Essays on Current Research 7th Series, Nuffield Provincial Hospitals Trust, Oxford University Press, London.

Carter E 1981 Ready for home? Nursing Times 77(19): 826-829.

Cartwright A 1964 Human relations and hospital care. Routledge & Kegan Paul, London.

Chambers LW, Woodward CA, Dok C 1980 Guide to health needs assessment: a critique of available sources of health and health care information. Department of Clinical Epidemiology and Biostatistics, McMaster University, Hamilton, Ontario.

Chelf JH, Deshler AMB, Theimann KMB, Dose AM, Quella SK, Hillman S 2002 Learning and support preferences of adult patients with cancer at a comprehensive cancer center. Oncology Nursing Forum 29(5): 863-7..

Dodge JS 1969 Factors related to patients' perceptions of their cognitive needs. Nursing Research 18(6): 502-513.

Dodge JS 1972 What patients should be told: patients' and nurses' beliefs. American Journal of Nursing 72(10): 1852-1854.

Eardley A, Davis F, Wakefield J 1975 Health education by chance: the unmet needs of patients in hospital and after. International Journal of Health Education 18(1): 19-25.

Emmerson C, Frayne C, Goodman A 2002 How much would it cost to increase UK health spending to the European Union average? Briefing Note No. 21. Institute for Fiscal Studies, London.

Faulkner A 1980 Communication and the nurse: Nursing Times 76(21) Occasional paper: 93-95

Faulkner A 1981 Aye there's the rub. Nursing Times 77(8): 332-336.

Greene JY, Weinberger M, Mamlin JJ 1980 Patient attitude towards health care: expectation of primary care in a clinical setting. Social Service and Medicine Oxford 14a(2): 133-138.

Hayward J 1975 Information: a prescription against pain. Royal College of Nursing, London.

Held E, Mygind K, Wolff C, Gyntelberg F, Agner T 2002 Prevention of work related skin problems: an intervention study in wet work employees. Occupational & Environmental Medicine 59(8): 556-61.

Henshaw L 2001 The impact of class position on women's experience of receiving health education information whilst in hospital. Health Education Journal. 60(3): 241-55.

Hugh-Jones P, Tansor AR, Whitby C 1964 Patients' view of admission to a London teaching hospital. British Medical Journal 2(5410): 661-664.

Katz M L, Smith-Whitley K, Ruzek SB, Ohene-Frempong K 2002 Knowledge of stroke risk, signs of stroke, and the need for stroke education among children with sickle cell disease and their caregivers. Ethnicity & Health 7(2): 115-23.

Kiger AM 1992 Pictures in their minds: an analysis of student nurses' images of nursing. Unpublished PhD thesis, University of Edinburgh.

Kiger AM 1993 Accord and discord in student nurses' images of nursing. Journal of Nursing Education 32(7): 309-317.

Kiger AM 1994 Student nurses' involvement with death: the image and the experience. Journal of Advanced Nursing 20: 679-686.

Koivula M, Paunonen-Ilmonen M, Tarkka MT, Tarkka M, Laippala P 2002 Social support and its relation to fear and anxiety in patients awaiting coronary artery bypass grafting. Journal of Clinical Nursing 11(5): 622-33.

Krathwohl DK, Bloom BS, Masia BB 1964 Taxonomy of educational objectives, handbook II: affective domain. David McKay, New York.

Ley P, Spelman MS 1967 Communicating with the patient. Staples Press, London.

Linehan DT 1966 What does the patient want to know? American Journal of Nursing 66(5): 1066-1070.

McIntosh J 1976 Patients' awareness and desire for information about diagnosed but undisclosed malignant disease. Lancet ii: 300-303.

Marsh N 1979 The patient needs to talk. Nursing Mirror 148(26): 16-18.

Maslow A 1954 Motivation and personality. Harper & Row, New York.

Melia K 1981 Student nurses' accounts of their work and training: a qualitative analysis. Unpublished Doctoral dissertation, University of Edinburgh.

Melia K 1987 Learning and working: the occupational socialization of nurses. Tavistock, London.

Mitchell M 2000 Psychological preparation for patients undergoing day surgery. Ambulatory Surgery. 8(1): 19-29.

Organisation for Economic Co-operation and Development (OECD) 2001 Health Data 2001 http://www.oecd.org/els/health/software Accessed April 20, 2003.

Office of Health Economics 1989 Compendium of health statistics 7th edn. Office of Health Economics, London.

Okun MA, Rice GE 2001 The effects of personal relevance of topic and information type on older adults' accurate recall of written medical passages about osteoarthritis. Journal of Aging & Health. 13(3): 410-29.

Pearson E 2001 A light at the end of the tunnel: An exploratory study of how patients cope with their emergency surgical event. Unpublished MSc Nursing dissertation, University of Aberdeen.

Pohl ML 1965 Teaching activities of the nursing practitioner. Nursing Research 14(1): 4-11.

Pratt L, Seligmann A, Reader G 1957 Physicians' view on the level of medical information among patients. American Journal of Public Health 47(10): 1277-1283.

Raphael W 1977 Patients and their hospitals. King Edward's Hospital Fund, London.

Redman BK 1971 Patient education as a function of nursing practice. Nursing Clinics of North America 6: 573-580.

Redman BK 1975 Guidelines for quality of care in patient education. Canadian Nurse 71: 19-21.

Reynolds M 1978 No news is bad news: patients' views about communication in hospital. British Medical Journal 1(6128): 1674-1676.

Ryan P, Lauver DR 2002 The efficacy of tailored intervention. Journal of Nursing Scholarship 34(4): 331-7.

Samson CD, Wakefield J, Pinnock KM 1971 Choice or chance? How women come to have a cytotest done by the family doctor. International Journal of Health Education 14(2): 127-138.

Sims P 1977 The dental habits dental knowledge and dental attitudes of Southend teenagers 1975. Public Health 91(4): 189-201.

Skipper JK, Tagliacozzo DL, Mauksch HO 1964 What communication means to patients. American Journal of Nursing 64(4): 101-103.

Smith JP 1979 The challenge of health education for nurses in the 1980s. Journal of Advanced Nursing 4: 531-543.

Webster ME 1981 Communication with dying patients. Nursing Times 77(23): 999-1002.

Young DS, Bekeris LG (1999) Paying for health care in the USA. Annals of Clinical Biochemistry 36(1): 1-9.

Yura H, Walsh MB 1988 The nursing process: assessing, planning, implementing, evaluating, 5th edn. Appleton & Lange, Norwalk Connecticut.

7 Planning: preparation for teaching

Once the patient's or client's health learning needs have been identified and analysed, the health teacher is ready to plan the teaching-learning activity. Again this fits well with the analogous stage of the nursing process.

THE MEANING OF PLANNING

In health teaching it is important for planning to be an active process, incorporating the identification of alternative ways to meet specified goals and decisions about the best way to achieve desired results. Planning should also involve the identification of possible pitfalls, and preparation for their avoidance. The prudent teacher will have plan B ready in case plan A fails. Planning is about thinking things through: it requires imagination and lateral, as well as logical, thinking.

Planning, therefore, is a process which directs the health teacher and health learner toward certain actions which will facilitate learning.

WHO PLANS?

The person to be taught, and perhaps the relatives, as well as the relevant health care professionals, should be involved in planning for health teaching. Doctors, nurses, and other professionals have separate though complementary roles to play. In patient education the doctor may, in some circumstances, be required to indicate a willingness to have teaching or information-giving carried out.

FIGURE 7.1   *Progression of client and health teacher roles. Adapted from Ewing 1984*

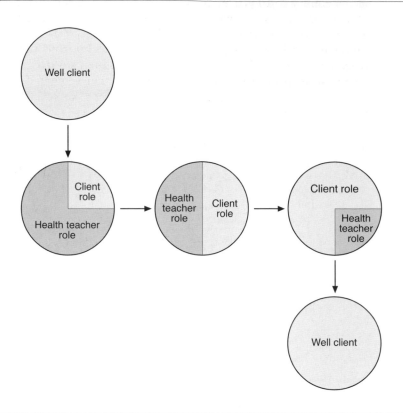

Differences in medical and nursing roles in health education are often not spelled out and may depend largely upon custom and usage, or 'tradition'. The doctor may expect, or be expected, to assess the person's information needs in relation to such aspects as diagnosis, investigations and treatment, and will usually assume responsibility for communicating most if not all of this information to the person. The nurse carries out a complementary process of assessing needs, often paying particular attention to affective and psychomotor needs as well as cognitive needs. The nurse will be concerned to weigh the person's needs against his or her ability and willingness to learn, and part of the planning activity may be related to determining how the doctor's instructions about information to be communicated may be interpreted in the individual's best interest.

Occasionally there is a disparity between the views of the doctor and the nurse as to what a patient should be told. This may happen, for example, in the case of a person with a terminal diagnosis or cancer. If the nurse believes that the doctor's decision about what is to be divulged to the patient will limit the teaching plan in a way that does not meet the patient's needs, then negotiation between the nurse and the doctor is needed.

The client's participation in planning is encouraged to the extent that is possible for the individual. Most critically ill people will not have the desire, and may not be able, to be involved. Even in these cases, the nurse has a responsibility to convey to the client or the family what is being planned and why. This allows for a degree of participation and control on the part of the ill person. The professional health teacher's ultimate goal is that the client become self-motivated and self-caring about his or her health; thus the planning phase in teaching should address short-term and long-term goals in which the nurse's role is seen to decrease as a result of goal achievement. Figure 7.1 illustrates how this can happen. The client role can be defined more broadly in the case of the severely ill or comatose person to include the family or significant others. These are the people who have knowledge of the individual and are likely to be able to describe the type of person he or she is, what he or she likes or doesn't like and so on. Their role in decision-making and planning, like the nurse's, should normally decrease as the client becomes more able to participate.

In the case of clients who are less ill, their participation should be sought throughout the process of planning. They will have been consulted in the information-gathering stage, and perhaps again when that information is being analysed. They should share in setting the learning goals and should have input into the plan for reaching those goals. The whole process will be more effective if the patient or client feels a sense of ownership and does not feel it is being imposed.

In instances of health teaching to healthy individuals, those individuals can often be taken into the planning process from the outset. When this involves group teaching, such as when the nurse is invited to do a teaching session, the programme organizer may take part in the planning.

THE MECHANICS OF PLANNING

The planning process involves checking the prioritizing that was carried out at the end of the assessment phase, setting learning objectives, and deciding on the teaching that will achieve the objectives. The latter is accomplished by considering methods and learning aids, the environment and the teacher's capabilities. Lastly, the client's motivation level and readiness to learn have to be assessed and encouraged.

Learning priorities

In the assessment phase, learning priorities are established by deciding which items are most important and have to be attended to first. Categorizations such as Maslow's (1954) hierarchy of needs or Redman's (1975) guidelines are useful tools for prioritizing, as suggested in Chapter 6. In the planning phase other aspects of prioritizing can be considered.

Learning needs have to be separated from other care needs, but they should be adapted to them and complement them. Obviously, only essential nursing can be carried out in a situation that is life-threatening or demands speedy action. For a person suffering from acute bronchitis, for example, the priority must be to relieve breathlessness. Subsequently, however, it may be appropriate to include teaching aimed at reducing smoking as one part of nursing intervention. In less acute situations, the challenge is to identify the sequence of teaching most likely to be useful to the individual. Should explanations be given before new skills are tried? Or will it be better for the client to experiment first and address the details later? Such questions can only be answered in the light of individual circumstances and there is no single formula for getting things right.

In health teaching, it is often appropriate to identify short- and long-term goals and plan accordingly. For example, for a patient in hospital, it may be appropriate to concentrate only on short-term goals during the period of hospitalization, and to save the long-term goals for attention after discharge. The nurse then has to decide in which areas health teaching is most needed. Again, this must be considered in conjunction with the client, because he or she will be able to verbalize a personal view of which long-term goals he or she is capable of achieving outside of hospital. This also implies the importance of liaison with other health professionals who may be responsible for after-care, which in turn implies the importance of making a written plan and keeping a record of implementation and progress. Here again the patient or client may be an active participant. Recording need not be seen as solely the province of the health professional.

The objectives approach to planning

Specifying objectives is one way of establishing the basis for an organized teaching plan. The use of objectives has its basis in the behaviourist school of educational psychology and has been much in favour as an essential component in instructional design for many years (Romiszowski 1981; Rowntree 1982; Laurillard 1993; Dean & Kenworthy 2000; Bastable 2003). Such a view accepts the premise that the only real evidence of learning is a change in behaviour. That being accepted, it follows that stating the outcomes of learning in terms of specified behaviours makes it possible to ascertain whether that learning has taken place or not. This, of course, ignores the possibility that some individuals, even if they have 'learned', will choose not to carry out the specified behaviour, thus exercising their right to autonomy. For such reasons, some educationalists have suggested that the objectives approach is too limiting. Ramsden (1992), for example, has said that 'learning is best conceptualized as a change in the way in which people understand the world around them, rather than as a quantitative accretion of facts and procedures' (p. 82). Such a view implies a need for a different type of outcome specification, but this will be addressed later. Meantime it is worth giving attention to the objectives approach, because it has much to offer that may be appropriate for health teaching activities geared to the needs of individuals.

The process of writing objectives can help to clarify purpose, establish what content is relevant and realistic, and identify suitable teaching methods. Additionally, if objectives are well written they provide a means to evaluate teaching. Clarifying the purpose of teaching and establishing what content will be relevant are often the most difficult parts of the teaching process. In any health teaching there will be a small central core of knowledge and skills which are essential for the individual to master. Beyond that are many areas which may or may not need to be included in order to help the individual understand the information or develop the needed skills. The extent and nature of that extra material varies, as some people need more help to understand things than do others, and the background knowledge and experience individuals bring to the learning situation are of almost infinite variety.

Beyond the range of things needed to aid understanding are the many items of interest which could be included in a teaching session. Adding items of interest is an important part of planning for teaching because interest is a stimulus to motivation. There is always the temptation, however, to add the interest items in response to the teacher's need for stimulation as much as to the learner's needs. Writing objectives for teaching helps to clarify whose needs are being met by the teaching plan.

In everyday use, the words 'aim' and 'objective' are interchangeable. When applied to educational planning, however, they take on particular meanings. Educationalists use the term 'aim' to denote a broad statement of the intention of the learning activity, often expressed from the teacher's viewpoint. An example of an aim might be: 'To teach Mr Jones to perform insulin injection accurately and safely' or 'To enable a group of healthy women to understand the value of routine cervical screening'.

The term 'objective', on the other hand, refers to a carefully worded statement which precisely identifies the behaviour the learner is expected to achieve. In order to emphasize that the term has precise meaning, some educationalists apply the adjectives 'instructional' or 'behavioural' to objectives. Mager (1962) described three main characteristics of a behavioural objective:

1. It is stated in learner terms.
2. It describes terminal behaviour.
3. It has in-built evaluation.

Stating objectives in terms of the learner

An objective should state what the teaching is intended to accomplish, what the learner will be expected to do or display knowledge of, as a result of the teaching. Writing an objective in learner, rather than teacher, terms provides a challenge in relation to evaluation of the lesson. Consider the differences between the ways the goal of teaching is stated in these two examples:

Objective A: The learner will describe the role of sugar in the formation of dental caries.

Objective B: The teacher will outline the role of sugar in the formation of dental caries.

The goal in objective B may be met if the teacher merely talks for an allotted time, whereas there is no way to be sure the goal in objective A has been met without testing the learner in some way. In Mager's terms, the second 'objective' is not a learning objective. It is merely a statement of the teacher's intended activity, and may not correlate with whether the learner has learned anything.

So the first rule in writing objectives is to express them in terms of the learner, showing what he or she will be able to do as a result of the teaching-learning activity.

Describing the learner's terminal behaviour

Objective A in the example above is a statement about the learner's terminal behaviour, that is, what she will be able to do after teaching. In this case, she will be able to describe something. Useful description of terminal behaviour largely depends on using the right verb. In the example given, the word 'describe' was used, which means that the objective, as stated, specified action which is capable of being observed. Some verbs specify 'action' which is not directly observable. Again, contrast the two objectives stated below:

Objective A: The learner will describe the role of sugar in the formation of dental caries.

Objective B: The learner will know about the role of sugar in the formation of dental caries.

It is impossible to observe 'knowing'. The learner will have to be asked to do something additional to demonstrate his knowledge. Describing, on the other hand, can be observed by hearing or reading the learner's description, so 'describe' is a better verb than 'know' to use in defining the terminal behaviour. Thus the first example is worded more effectively than the second because it enables the teacher to ascertain that learning has occurred. So the second rule when writing objectives is to choose language which designates learner actions that are capable of direct observation.

Building in evaluation

An objective should be stated in terms of observable learner behaviour and should be capable of evaluation. This means that somewhere within the objective there should be an indication of the standard that will be used to judge the learner's performance, and the conditions under which it will be observed. In the example given above, the person is expected to be able to describe the role of sugar in the formation of dental caries, but there is no indication of how detailed or accurate the description needs to be, or how it will be performed. As it stands, the objective does not specify these aspects, so it is a less useful statement of educational intent than it might be. A third rule in writing objectives, then, is to ensure that each objective identifies the criteria required for successful performance of the terminal behaviour.

In the instance given above, if a fairly simple description of the role of sugar is all that is required, then it would be easy to specify the nature, standard, and conditions of performance required of the learner by indicating the components of knowledge and how these will be displayed. The objective might be written thus:

Objective: When questioned, the learner will, by responding orally:
- describe the role of sugar in the formation of dental caries, including:
  - the relationship between the metabolism of sugar in the mouth and the formation of plaque
  - the effects of plaque on tooth enamel
- explain the relationship between increased sugar intake and the formation of plaque.

For most health teaching this is likely to be a satisfactory way of identifying evaluation criteria. Sometimes, however, more detailed knowledge is required,

TABLE 7.1	Cognitive and affective learning objectives in teaching the role of sugar in dental caries

Objectives	Level of achievement
After teaching the learner will:	
Cognitive learning	
1. Identify sucrose as the sugar most implicated in dental caries.	Knowledge
2. Describe the composition of plaque.	Knowledge
3. Recount at least one experiment demonstrating the production of acid after sugar ingestion.	Knowledge
4. Identify patterns of sugar ingestion most likely to contribute to the development of caries.	Application
5. Name three foods with high and three foods with low sucrose content.	Comprehension
Affective learning	
1. Hold the attitude that avoiding dental caries is worth the self-denial involved in sugar regulation.	Valuing
2. Believe that dental caries is preventable.	Valuing
3. Believe that preventing dental caries is desirable.	Valuing
4. Believe that personal efforts will make an impact on the prevention of dental caries.	Valuing
5. Regulate sugar intake to minimize acid attack on tooth enamel.	Characterization

perhaps because the person has to grasp an understanding of a complex disease process or because the individual is especially curious about details and causation. In such an instance, a single global objective may have to be replaced by a more detailed series of objectives, distinguished in relation to the cognitive, affective and psychomotor learning required. In the dental health example outlined earlier, there are cognitive and affective learning objectives which might be written as shown in Table 7.1. (Note that the 'valuing' objectives are not capable of being observed as behaviours.)

Writing separate objectives for cognitive, affective and psychomotor learning completes the analysis of the educational task. In the example above, an appropriate change in behaviour based on the cognitive learning will depend on the person's attitude. The attitude will have to be supported by a cluster of beliefs about the benefits and probability of prevention. Once the desired level of achievement is specified in each learning domain, it can be seen that the affective learning desired requires the highest level of learning. Such detailed analysis of objectives raises questions about the reactions and learning capabilities of the individual, and it becomes obvious that it will be essential to involve the person him- or herself in the analysis and planning tasks. Objectives for sugar regulation, for instance, can only be set realistically in the light of what the individual contracts to do. Ideally, sweet things between meals should be avoided completely and there should be a move from highly refined sugar in the diet to other sugars and sweeteners. For some people this will require only minimal adjustment. Others may opt to begin by cutting out sweets between meals or by contracting to reduce sweet consumption while watching television. This example illustrates the danger of pressing on regardless, in pursuit of well-written objectives. Though there are useful rules, they should be applied to aid the thinking processes surrounding the planning of teaching, rather than being blindly followed.

Writing objectives can be difficult, but the benefits are that the purpose of teaching may become clarified, and the means of evaluation identified. If teacher and learner alike have a clear idea of what is to be accomplished then it will be possible to assess what is being achieved. One way to clarify purpose is to try to be as unambiguous as possible in stating the standard of performance that will be required of the learner.

Limitations of behavioural objectives

As was alluded to above, the use of behavioural objectives is sometimes criticized on the grounds that they may lead to inflexibility in teaching. Another criticism is that by concentrating on what is measurable, they limit the view of what it is possible to teach and, more importantly, to learn. These potential dangers are particularly likely to be damaging in health teaching, since involving the learner actively in the process necessitates a wide and flexible approach. The benefits related to the clarification of teaching purpose may mean that the advantages of well-written objectives will outweigh the disadvantages, as long as objectives are used as an analytic tool in the planning process and not as an end in themselves. They can be used as a guide rather than as a strict prescription.

Another potential disadvantage is the time required to prepare the detail necessary for well-written objectives. One thing that can be said in mitigation here is that after practising the preparation of objectives, the process may be internalized to the extent that it is used (though not formally written out) even in brief instances of on-the-spot teaching.

Planning for flexibility: the outcomes approach

There is considerable confusion in some of the terminology used in education, and although educationalists have defined their meaning of the term 'objectives' quite precisely, the same cannot be said with respect to approaches that do not use objectives. In certain spheres of health education and health promotion, notably within community education and youth work, the objectives approach has found less favour than it has had in mainstream educational spheres. The reasons for this have been mentioned in the discussion in the previous section.

One way of designating a non-objectives-based approach is to use the phrase 'learning outcomes'. A problem with this terminology, however, is that its use is inconsistent and therefore ambiguous. It is sometimes used to refer to the 'competencies' that are assessed for NVQs and SVQs (National Vocational Qualifications and Scottish Vocational Qualifications) in the UK. This is not the sense that is very useful for health educators, because it relates to the performance of specific skills and therefore does not encompass the sorts of goals or intentions that health educators find missing in the objectives approach.

Another meaning sometimes implied by the term 'learning outcomes' is the one that, for health educators, is a potentially useful adjunct to the objectives approach. This sense attributes a broader and more fluid meaning to the process and goals of education.

Health educators sometimes want to allow a teaching–learning episode to develop according to its own direction and momentum. This might be the case, for example, in a session with teenagers about sexuality and relationships. Whereas objectives may be helpful in the planning, they cannot account for everything that might be accomplished, and if followed strictly they may not allow adequate flexibility. Thus the 'outcomes of learning' may go beyond what is planned in the objectives. In addition, the longer-term dimension of outcomes can be more difficult to pin down and describe as objectives than are the shorter-term aspects that are easily expressed as objectives. In the same example, if the learning about relationships is effective, the young people may acquire values and attitudes that influence their lives in a multitude of ways for many years. So it would be useful to have a term that could be used as a label for these other dimensions of the outcomes of learning, and one whose meaning was generally agreed upon.

This section was headed 'the outcomes approach', which was as near the mark as any other terminology that could be found. In fact, the phrase 'outcomes of learning' may be more suitable than 'learning outcomes'. There is a fine semantic difference, but 'outcomes of learning' does seem to imply greater breadth and potentially greater diversity.

A question that might be asked at this point is, 'If we are talking about learning outcomes, and their breadth and diversity, what do these have to do with planning?' This is a valid question, as the outcomes follow the learning, and the breadth and diversity are the very things the health teacher is trying not to plan for prescriptively. The answer may be that in the planning, the health teacher needs to allow leeway for the unanticipated, and should sometimes be willing to risk relying on his or her expert intuition. It may be fair to say that although one may not be able to plan flexibility, one can plan *for* flexibility.

PREPARING TO TEACH

When learning objectives (or anticipated outcomes) have been formulated, the participants to the teaching–learning process decide on the methods, aids and environmental requirements that will enable those objectives to become operational. Information relevant to this decision-making is provided in Chapters 3 and 4. At this point, general comments only are made concerning these aspects.

Choosing a method of teaching

If objectives are specified in cognitive, affective and psychomotor terms, this helps to clarify the type of teaching needed. Consider the cognitive and affective objectives in the dental health example quoted earlier. The cognitive objectives may be met by some didactic teaching: a leaflet might do, provided it is at the right reading level, and assuming the person has no undue suspicion of scientific evidence. The affective objectives present a different challenge. Here the learner needs to have a chance to explore beliefs and test them with others. Less didactic teaching is needed. The person will either need a chance to challenge the nurse's position on self-denial of sugar or, ideally, be helped to examine the issue with a group of other learners.

Choosing aids to enhance learning

The purpose of a learning aid should be to facilitate learning in an identified way, not simply to fill up time or to embellish the teaching session. The aid should enhance rather than merely duplicate any factual information. If it introduces unnecessary extra material which is likely to confuse, it should be abandoned.

If audiovisual aids are to be used it is important to check that equipment will operate as anticipated. The only way to do this is to rehearse its use: make sure slides are in sequence and will project the right way up; rehearse the operation of the slide or overhead projector and check that projected material can be seen adequately from the learner's viewpoint; locate electric points and be sure there is a screen in place; if computer projection (e.g. 'Powerpoint') is to be used, be sure all necessary equipment and connectors are present – and so on. These preparations should be done in advance, as it is deterimental to the flow of the session and the effectiveness of the presentation if the equipment fails to function properly or the teacher is unable to operate it readily.

Planning the teaching–learning environment

Some aspects of the teaching–learning environment may be difficult to control. A hospital ward can be noisy, possibly with upsetting activities going on, and there may be a lack of privacy; a home can be busy with children watching television, telephones and doorbells ringing. It is important to do as much as possible to minimize the intrusive effects of such factors. In hospital, there may be a side ward or day room available, or perhaps it would help to screen the bed. In the home, it may be possible to find quiet activities for the children, and perhaps another room to go into from which they can still be seen. It will help to have the opportunity to sit down comfortably in relaxed surroundings when very personal concerns are to be discussed.

The psychological setting is as important as the physical setting. The learner needs to feel confident that the teacher intends to communicate clearly and will give undivided attention to the person and the learning activity. In group settings it may be useful to arrange furniture so that people can see each other. That way no one feels peripheral to the activity, and no hierarchy is established by virtue of positioning. In some situations a cup of tea or coffee may ease the initial moments and give groups of relative strangers the opportunity to relax together before the session begins.

Planning for teacher involvement

Some kinds of teaching are more demanding than others. If attitudes and beliefs are to be examined, the nurse needs to consider his or her own before the session. If feelings are to be explored it is advisable to consider possible personal reactions and the extent to which it will be, both personally and pro-

BOX 7.1	*Self-exploration check list for use in planning teaching*

- What are my values and attitudes related to this aspect of health/health care?
- How do I feel about interacting with this person? Can I respect him? Will I be able to accept his views? Do I intend to act as informant, teacher, persuader or enabler?
- Are there differences of language, age and social class? Can anything be done about them?
- Is what I do congruent with what I advise? Need it be congruent?

fessionally, acceptable and possible to share feelings with someone else who may have established role expectations as client or patient. The planned teaching should neither exceed the capabilities nor conflict with sincerely held convictions of the teacher concerned. Box 7.1 illustrates a useful self-check list. Where there is a potential problem of values conflict it may be wiser for another nurse to take over teaching in a given area or with a particular person.

Planning for client involvement

The level of motivation and state of readiness of the client will have been assessed and will have an impact on planning. The client who has just had a myocardial infarction may be well motivated to learn how to avoid further cardiac incidents by reducing the stress he has been experiencing, stopping smoking, taking regular exercise and maintaining his weight at an appropriate level. However, his readiness to learn may initially be complicated by factors such as fear and pain. The health teacher needs to keep these factors in mind when planning the teaching sessions.

In some cases a reluctance to learn may be overcome by encouraging a commitment of some sort – what is often referred to as a learning contract. Such contracts can be oral or written, formal or informal, depending on circumstances. They entail an agreement between the teacher and the learner as to what the learning needs and goals are, how they are to be addressed, including how responsibility is shared between the two parties, and what will count as success. Contracts need to be reviewed regularly to assess progress, to change objectives if necessary as more data collection occurs and to remind both participants of their commitment. In situations where these tasks are carried out with written contracts, the client or patient should always have his or her own copy to review. In addition to its practical purpose, this has the effect of affirming the shared ownership of the process.

At this point in planning, it is also wise to reflect on the information gathered about the client's past learning experiences and the ways in which, as reported by the client, he or she learns best. For instance, a learner who says he has always had difficulty learning concepts may be describing an inability to learn from a holist-style presentation (see Chapter 3), and his preferred approach may be a serialist one. To be successful, the teaching activity will need to be planned according to this style preference, unless it is appropriate for one of the learning aims to be the fostering of versatility of learning style.

ACTIVITY 7.1

Consider the health learning needs you identified for your 'learner' in Activity 6.1. Decide what you would address in a first teaching episode with this person. In making this decision, you will need to take account of the priorities you assigned to the person's various health learning needs, and you will also need to consider the person's own views on this. It is essential that you have the learner's agreement about the need and the value of learning, if he or she is to be a willing learner.

Once you have identified a focus for the teaching activity, try planning the activity. What would your aim be, as the health teacher? Try writing a set of objectives for the session. Remember to state them using verbs that denote observable behaviour (e.g. through acting, speaking or writing). Do you encounter any difficulties with this? Does the nature of the needed learning lend itself to planning by objectives? If not, what alternative planning approach would you take?

Now that you know broadly where your session is heading, there are a number of other decisions to be made. What would be an appropriate setting for the teaching–learning activity? What method(s) would you use? Would any audiovisual aids be helpful? How would you ensure that your own knowledge and understanding were sufficient for the teaching?

Now try writing an outline plan for your teaching session. How long would it take? How would you divide up the time? What would your own role be, and what participation would you want from your learner?

Finally, explain what you would hope your learner would know, believe, and/or be able to do as a result of your teaching-learning session.

THE TEACHING PLAN

Teaching plans are not always written down. A mental check list or plan of action may be all that is needed in some instances, and has the advantage of saving time in documentation. It is certainly more important to make a plan than to be in possession of a written sheet purporting to be a plan. As with other aspects of the nursing process, if the paper work inhibits the care or teaching, it is being overdone. Nonetheless, written plans can often be useful, especially in complex teaching, since the very act of writing the plan may trigger further analysis and planning. Written plans also provide reminders for action, a framework for documentation and evaluation of teaching, and serve as a communication device to other involved professionals.

Written teaching plans will vary, but in general, certain key elements should be included:

- A description of the learner(s)
- A list of prioritized learning needs
- A statement of objectives or intended learning outcomes
- A note of aids and barriers to learning
- An outline of content
- An indication of sequence
- A description of teaching method

- Notes on the use of teaching aids
- Notes on environmental preparation
- Actual outcome (evaluation notes).

A potential problem with teaching plans is that they may be poorly utilized. They must be written in clear concise language so that fellow health teachers readily comprehend their intent. Strict adherence to a plan may reduce flexibility with changing needs. The procedure for using the plan, therefore, should encourage constant re-assessment of needs, priorities and teaching actions. By each having a copy of the plan and reviewing it and referring to it, both the health learner and teacher can measure progress and be accountable.

Example of a teaching plan

In the case shown in Box 7.2, only parts of the plan are fully developed. It is acknowledged that clients newly diagnosed as having diabetes mellitus would have a number of other learning needs which are not presented here.

Much health teaching that is carried out by nurses in hospital is only the first stage of a much longer undertaking. Diabetic education is a good example: the hospital nurse can only begin a process which will continue throughout the rest of the person's life. Many of the goals will not be reached until long after discharge from hospital. For evaluation purposes, it is therefore important to distinguish between short- and long-term goals. The immediate concerns are whether the patient is learning the things it is appropriate to learn at this stage, and whether the teaching is being done in the most helpful way. In addition to using the formal mechanisms of the teaching plan and the documentation of results of care, an essential element in assessing the effectiveness of teaching is simply asking the patient. As a partner in the teaching–learning process, and as its intended beneficiary, his or her view is arguably the most important. Provision for this step should also be included in the planning.

Once planning has concluded, action is taken (see Figure 7.2 for the continuous nature of the teaching–learning process) and teaching occurs.

ACTIVITY 7.2

Refer back to your notes on Activity 6.2. Once again, imagine how you would actually go about planning the teaching session. In this case, the timing and the setting are planned for you – you have no real choice. However, you still need to go through the other steps in planning.

For the topic you selected, decide whether an objectives approach or some other approach would be appropriate. Write an outline of the content you would include. What method(s) would you use in presenting your topic? What would your role be, and how would you expect the children to participate? In this case, because they are young and they are not ill, you may have to give a bit of extra thought to how you will encourage their interest and motivation. You may need to persuade them of the relevance of the topic to themselves and their lives. How will you plan to do this? Would any audiovisual aids be appropriate?

What would you hope to have achieved with the children by the end of the session? That is, how would their behaviour, skills and/or attitudes have changed as a result of your teaching?

BOX 7.2	*Example of a teaching plan*

Name: *Ann Smith*   Age: *18*   Marital Status: *Single*   Date: *26 March 2003*

Address: *University residence*

Occupation: *1st year university student, studying philosophy*

Religion: *Non-practising*

Next of kin: *Mother – Mrs J Smith*   Address: *City, 200 miles away*

Diagnosis: *Diabetes mellitus, is aware of diagnosis*

Previous medical history: *Reports 'I've never been sick before except for the odd cold'*

Learning needs		**Priority**
1.	To develop self-care knowledge and skills to prevent complications and optimize health	Short term
2.	To accept that regulation of blood sugar will have to become a conscious aspect of lifestyle	Longer term

Aids or barriers to learning

Quick to grasp detail. Appears confident

Environmental concerns

Prefers one-to-one sessions with privacy

TEACHING PLAN

Learning need	*Objectives – with learning the client will:*	*Teaching action (methods and aids)*
1. To develop self-care skills to prevent complications and optimize health	1a. Describe the pathophysiology of diabetes: – cause – complications – treatment	Booklets x 2 Discussion
	1b. Correctly test urine: – relate results to status of diabetes	Explanation Demonstration Return demonstration Supervised practice
	1c. Choose correct insulin: – type and strength – action	Work with vials Drug information

BOX 7.2 cont	Example of a teaching plan

Learning need	Objectives – with learning the client will:	Teaching action (methods and aids)
	1d. Correctly calculate dosage: – relate to acidosis and hypoglycaemia	Explanation Supervised practice
	1e. Safely administer injections: – correct technique – review aspects of safety	Explanation Demonstration Return demonstration Supervised practice
	1f. Discuss the relationship of diet to diabetes: – choose appropriate foods and explain their relevance	Refer to dietician Use menu sheets
	1g. Discuss the relationship of exercise to diabetes	Booklets Discussion Use case examples
	1h. Explain reasons for special care: of feet, eyes, skin, minor illnesses	Booklets

Need and objective	Dates of teaching	Evaluation date	Notes (initialled)
1a.	26/3/03	26/3/03	Appeared eager to learn. Asked questions. Would like more than booklets. One of British Diabetic Association suggested books given. (LC)
	28/3/03	29/3/03	Seems to feel overwhelmed by all the facts on diabetes. Is able to correctly identify cause and complications of condition but is having difficulty relating how the treatment works. Introduced to another client with diabetes who felt same way when first learning. (LKH)
	28/3/03	2/4/03	Is proud to be able to explain disease process. Says 'Mary [fellow patient] told me I would be learning all my life about diabetes and all that I learned would help me to feel well.' (LKH)

FIGURE 7.2   *The planning process*

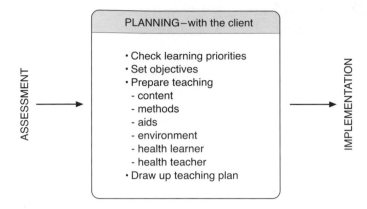

REFERENCES

Bastable SB 2003 Nurse as educator: Principles of teaching and learning for nursing practice, 2nd edn. Jones and Bartlett Publishers, Sudbury, Massachusetts.

Dean J, Kenworthy N 2000 The principles of teaching. In: Nicklin P J & Kenworthy N, Teaching and assessing in nursing practice: an experiential approach. Ballière Tindall in association with the Royal College of Nursing, Edinburgh.

Ewing G 1984 A study of the post-operative nursing care of stoma patients during appliance changes. Unpublished doctoral dissertation, University of Edinburgh.

Laurillard D 1993 Rethinking university teaching: a framework for the effective use of educational technology. Routledge, London.

Mager RF 1962 Preparing instructional objectives. Fearon, Palo Alto California.

Maslow A 1954 Motivation and personality. Harper & Row, New York.

Ramsden P 1992 Learning to teach in higher education. Routledge, London.

Redman BK 1975 Guidelines for quality of care in patient education. Canadian Nurse 71: 19-21.

Romiszowski AJ 1981 Designing instructional systems: decision making in course planning and curriculum design. Kogan Page, London.

Rowntree D 1982 Educational technology in curriculum development, 2nd edn. Harper & Row, London.

8 Implementing teaching plans

The implementation phase of the teaching–learning process activates the joint plans made by the health teacher and the learner. The aim of health teaching is the achievement of the goals that were defined in the planning stage. It is in the implementation phase that the nurse uses his or her theory base and skills actively, creatively and intelligently to help the client to learn about his or her health behaviour. This phase is demanding for the health teacher, who has to interact intentionally and effectively.

In this chapter, examples are presented to illustrate the process that occurs in health teaching. Each has a dynamic development which acknowledges that the phases of the teaching–learning process are continuous and interactive. None of the examples represents an actual situation, but each has been chosen to reflect realistic experiences in health teaching.

EXAMPLE 1: STOMA APPLIANCE MANAGEMENT

Assessment

PERSONAL DATA
Name: *Mr Jack Windsor*
Address: *121 Rue Road, Edinburgh*
Occupation: *Secondary school science teacher*
Marital Status: *Married, 2 children ages 4 and 6*
Religion: *Non-practising*
Height: *190.5 cm*

Date: *27 March 2003*
DOB: *21 October 1958*
Telephone: *666 1101*

Weight: *79.5 kg*

Reason for contact: Client has a newly formed loop colostomy and needs help learning to care for it.

Diagnosis: Cancer of the rectum. Sigmoid loop colostomy performed 26 March 2003. Client was an emergency admission. No preoperative counselling or teaching was accomplished.

PHYSICAL ASSESSMENT

Mr Windsor is 1 day post-operation. He is a clean-looking, well-proportioned individual who appears to be in no distress. He looks his stated age of 44 years. He is sitting up in bed speaking to his wife as I approach. He has an intravenous line running into a brachial site on his left arm. He is located in a ward bed.

VITAL SIGNS

Temperature: oral, 37.2 degrees centigrade
Pulse: right radial site, 86 per minute, regular
Respiration: 26 per minute, regular
Blood pressure: right brachial site, sitting up in bed, 144/76 mmHg

Physician's notes on physical assessment reveal that Mr Windsor has been experiencing lower abdominal pain for some time but thought it was due to occupational stress. He also reported problems with constipation and abdominal distension. A physical examination revealed no other health deficits. He was admitted with lower abdominal pain experienced over a 24-hour period. Abdominal X-ray indicated a bowel obstruction and immediate surgery was planned.

PSYCHOSOCIAL ASSESSMENT

Mr Windsor is a married 44-year-old secondary school teacher with two young children. He has been working as a teacher for 12 years but has been at his present school for only 2 years, as principal teacher in the science department. He says, 'The job has been tough. There's a lot of responsibility and the school has a strong reputation for science teaching, which the headmaster would like to maintain.' Mrs Windsor reports that her husband's personality has changed since he took on the principal teacher position: 'He used to be easy-going, played with the children (4-year-old son, 6-year-old daughter) and planned the occasional night out with me. Now he never seems to be home and when he is he works.'

Mrs Windsor works part-time as a nurse at a nursing home. She enjoys this work and feels her wages help to pay for the bills. She organizes day care for the 4-year-old and has arranged her hours so that she is able to take the 6-year-old to and from school.

Both husband and wife are from Edinburgh and have a wide social network of friends and relatives about whom they say, 'We can count on them.'

The present situation is a shock to both of them. Mr Windsor refers to his stoma by waving his hand in the direction of his abdomen and saying, 'that thing'. Mrs Windsor refers to 'the operation'. The surgeon has told them that the colostomy will be temporary. The tumour was extensive and Mr Windsor would be referred to an oncologist for radiotherapy and possible chemotherapy to reduce the tumour prior to further surgery.

SUMMARY OF ASSESSMENT

Client's questions/comments:

'How will "this" affect my work?'

'I don't know what this means for travelling abroad in the future.'

'How long will I have this thing?'

Anticipated needs (research based):

Diagnosis – explained by surgeon, needs to be followed up at oncology

Treatment – needs to be explained by colorectal nurse/stoma care nurse

Investigations – doctor to explain, nurse to detail and ensure comprehension

Prognosis – surgeon explains uncertainty, pending outcome of treatment

Progress – individual previously healthy, non-smoker, moderate (3-4 beers/week) drinker, jogs (3 miles) daily; expected to recover physical stamina quickly. Anticipated hospital stay – 8 days

Self-care – should progress to complete self-care with stoma care nurse support.

Routine – to be learned

Aids/barriers to learning:

Aids. Well educated, Mr Windsor will be able to understand the discussions about his colostomy and learn self-care. As a science teacher, he is accustomed to using manual skill to set up experiments and this should help him to manipulate the equipment used in stoma appliance management. His wife's nursing skills may be helpful in the long term, but she has no experience of stoma care, and in any case, her own need for support must not be overlooked.

Barriers. The colostomy was not anticipated. Mr Windsor is still shocked by the outcome of the surgery. His wife, a significant person in his life, has not yet accepted the colostomy. His motivation to learn about self-care is low. He has expressed no curiosity as yet.

Date	Learning deficit:	Learning need:	Priority
27/3/03	Non-acceptance of colostomy due to suddenness of surgery	To understand the reasons for the formation of the colostomy	1
27/3/03	Does not know about the physical care of his colostomy due to inexperience	To learn the principles of care for his stoma	2

Planning

LEARNING NEED 1:

TO UNDERSTAND THE REASONS FOR THE RESULT OF SURGERY

The plan is to increase Mr Windsor's understanding of the reasons for the colostomy to help him towards acceptance of it. If he does not accept the results of surgery, he will not be motivated to learn about self-care.

Objectives: After teaching Mr Windsor will:

Cognitive learning	*Learning level*	*Teaching methods and aids*
1. Locate the site of his tumour in the large intestine (after 3 postoperative days)	Knowledge	Book diagrams One-to-one teaching
2. Discuss the functioning of the large intestine in relation to his colostomy (after 3 postoperative days)	Application	Discussion Diagrams to illustrate functioning of bowel
3. Identify when bowel movements in the colostomy are most likely to occur (after 3 postoperative days)	Application	Stoma care nurse to discuss effects of certain foods Leaflet from Colostomy Association

Affective learning	*Learning level*	*Teaching methods and aids*
1. Use proper terminology to refer to his colostomy (by discharge)	Receiving	Role model by using proper terminology consistently
2. Begin to discuss his feelings about the colostomy (by discharge)	Responding	Provide occasions for discussion, ensure privacy
3. Discuss how the colostomy will affect his teaching activities, jogging, sex life (within 6 weeks)	Valuing	Introduce him to an ostomy association and others successfully coping with ostomies. Provide opportunities and privacy for him to bring subjects up or to introduce subjects to him as possible areas of concern; include wife when possible; communicate this objective to community health nurse

LEARNING NEED 2:
TO LEARN THE PRINCIPLES OF CARE FOR HIS STOMA

The plan is to use a specific recording format designed by Ewing (1984) which summarizes on one sheet all pertinent detail about Mr Windsor and his progress in learning about the physical care of his stoma (see Figure 8.1). The listed guidelines are, in fact, the objectives for meeting the learning need of self-care, and the learning level will begin with Mr Windsor's being encouraged to develop appliance management or psychomotor skills (perception and set; see Chapter 3, Figure 3.3) and proceed to his using full self-care skills in which he is able to alter and innovate his use of stoma appliances (adaptation and origination). The nurse works through the helping methods with specific teaching strategies:

- *Acting*: by doing the appliance management
- *Teaching*: by demonstrating, explaining
- *Guiding*: by encouraging return demonstration
- *Supporting*: by watching, reinforcing, answering questions
- *Promoting self-care*: by praising, providing opportunity for independent care.

Implementation

Progress notes on Mr Windsor illustrate how he is progressing with his learning needs.

Date and time	Learning need	Nursing action and results
27/3/03 2:30 pm	1	After his wife left, I approached Mr Windsor, screened his bed and asked if I could check his colostomy site. I asked him how he felt about it and he replied, 'I feel a bit numb, as if it isn't quite true'. I asked him if he would look at the site so I could explain the words we use when describing it. He seemed to become interested and looked at the site with no apparent adverse reaction.
27/3/03 8:30 pm	1, 2	Colostomy appliance required changing. I explained to Mr Windsor the procedure and told him I would do the change but would tell him about each step. He responded, 'That is disgusting and smelly. You do what you want with it.' He sounded angry and refused to observe the appliance change procedure.

These notes indicate that Mr Windsor is not meeting his learning needs as yet. The nurse's approach must be consistent and understanding. In the second progress note the nurse commented on both learning needs because in reality they are inseparable. At this point the nurse could discuss Mr Windsor's needs with his wife and other members of the health care team, and the objectives and teaching plan may change to accommodate the situation. Or, because this is still the first postoperative day and Mr Windsor's reactions to his altered form of elimination are judged to be within normal limits, the nurse may continue with her teaching plan for another 24 hours.

FIGURE 8.1　Teaching plan for learning about stoma appliance management *Ewing 1984*

GUIDELINES	CARE DETAILS (DATE)						
Preparation of equipment	Tray						
Preparation of patient	Location Position Time						
Removal of old appliance	Method						
Skin care	Cleanser drying agent						
Skin protection	Intact Damaged Broken						
Selection of new appliance	Effluent–fluid firm Type Size						
Preparation of appliance	Method						
Application	Angle Accessories Closure						
Disposal	Method						

Helping method (enter code under date)
Acting–A
Teaching–T
Guiding–G
Supporting–S
Home care/ self care–SC

Developmental & environmental reminders:
Privacy
Uninterrupted care
Exposure of stoma only
Screening of patient
Terminology
Facial expression
No gloves

Patient details

Name: Jack Windsor

Date of birth: 21/10/62

Diagnosis: *Cancer of the rectum*

Operation: Laparotomy, loop colostomy 24/3/03

Type of stoma
ileostomy
colostomy ✓

Site of stoma
ileum
ascending colon
transverse colon
descending colon
sigmoid colon ✓

Form of stoma
end
loop ✓
double barrel

Length of stoma
spout
flush ✓
retracted

Physical condition
eyesight　no glasses
hearing　good
manual deformity　none
skin problems　none

Home conditions:
toilet facilities–inside, ground floor
means of disposal–city rubbish collection

COMMENTS

Works as manager in a hardware shop.
Lives with wife (works as secretary). 2 children live at home – daughter age 15 and son age 17. Another son age 20 in the army.
Allergic to some types of adhesive – doesn't know which.

ACTIVITY 8.1

With the permission of your 'volunteer learner' from Activity 6.1, try out the teaching plan you formulated in Activity 7.1. Make notes about your teaching in any format you like. You may like to consider the example cases described in this chapter to give you ideas about how you might make your notes. Keep these notes for use in a later exercise.

EXAMPLE 2: FEMALE SECONDARY SCHOOL STUDENTS AND MENSTRUATION

Pertinent data

Target group: class of 20 female secondary school students aged 12-13 years
Topic: menstruation
School: single-sex institution located in West Royal, a middle-class neighbourhood
Previous teaching: general introduction to the menarche at age 9-10, in a class on health
Time allowed by school authorities: three sessions of 40 minutes each

First session: 21 February 2003

The local health visitor is asked to conduct a health teaching session on menstruation for this class who, in a class with their registration teacher, related misinformation about their understanding of the menarche. The health visitor asked the school authorities for three class periods. The first session was planned as an assessment of the girls' knowledge and attitudes which would aid the organization of the other sessions. The initial learning deficits and related learning needs were discovered to be as follows:

Learning deficit	*Learning need*	*Priority*
1. Misinformed about menstruation	1. To understand the functioning of the body during menstruation	1
2. Attitudes about menstruation have been negative (e.g. 'the curse') due to misinformation and attitude expressed by initial sources of information	2. To explore their own attitudes about menstruation and how these have been formed	2

LEARNING NEED 1:
TO UNDERSTAND THE FUNCTIONING OF THE BODY DURING MEN-
STRUATION
Objectives: By the end of the session each student will be able to:

Cognitive	Learning level	Teaching strategies
1. Draw a diagram of the female reproductive system	Knowledge	Whole group: use board and coloured chalk; have handouts to label with organ names
2. Locate correctly the organs involved in menstruation	Knowledge	Whole group: use board and coloured chalk; have handouts to label with organ names
3. Explain the normal menstrual cycle	Comprehension	Whole group: use board and coloured chalk
4. Explain the hormonal changes occurring in menstruation	Knowledge	Use memory device to aid in remembering names of hormones
5. (For those who have started menstruating) Compare their own cycle with what has been presented	Application	One-to-one at end of session

LEARNING NEED 2:
TO EXPLORE THEIR OWN ATTITUDES ABOUT MENSTRUATION AND
HOW THESE HAVE BEEN FORMED

Objectives: By the end of the session each student will be able to:

Affective	Learning level	Teaching strategies
1. State her initial reaction to hearing that she will be a menstruating female	Responding	Small groups – four or five in each group. Set task of sharing their experience with one another. Report back to whole group
2. Discuss the things she has heard other people say about menstruation	Responding	Present list of myths about menstruation (see Box 8.1). Add student contributions, have students debate each myth
3. Name her primary informants	Responding	No strategy

| 4. Discuss others' ideas about menstruation in a non-judgemental fashion | Responding | Small group discussions with introduction about accepting others' experiences and feelings |
| 5. React to situations that can occur when female is menstruating | Responding | Have students list situations. Add to the list from Box 8.2 if necessary. Ask them to think of the worst that could happen |

BOX 8.1   *Myths about menstruation*

Women who are menstruating:

- Turn milk sour
- Stop bread rising
- Rust brass and iron
- Are unclean
- Must not exercise
- Must not wash their hair
- Student contribution
- Student contribution
- Student contribution
- Student contribution

BOX 8.2   *Situations that can occur during menstruation*

- Buying sanitary towels or tampons from a male assistant at the chemist's
- Leaking through layers of clothing
- Staying at a friend's house and having the family dog find your used sanitary towel in the rubbish bin
- Trying to explain to your new boyfriend that you are having menstrual pains and do not want to swim today
- Opening your bag in a crowd and having a tampon fall out
- Student suggestion
- Student suggestion
- Student suggestion

BOX 8.3	*Student interest list used to decide on topics*

Students to indicate by voting which topics are most popular:

- Feminine hygiene
- Toxic shock syndrome
- Premenstrual tension
- Menstruation and the pill
- Dysmenorrhoea
- Amenorrhoea
- Gynaecological examination
- Student suggestion
- Student suggestion
- Student suggestion

Progress notes: 21 February 2003

This first session was a bit chaotic. I decided to begin by being practical and helping them to learn about the anatomy and physiology of the menstrual cycle. They are a very keen group and proved quite able to grasp and remember facts. Six of the girls are already menstruating and two of these are very knowledgeable. They were able to contribute very well to this first part of the session. The last half of the session which explored attitudes was very noisy with much laughter and teasing. However, since the affective objectives were met, the second half appeared to be successful. Further assessment of the group was done in this session, and aids and barriers to learning were identified.

Aids. All the students have been achieving good results in school and their ability to participate in the fact-learning session was high. Some of the girls are menstruating and are willing to share their knowledge and/or experiences. They understand that this learning is important to them as females.

Barriers. The early adolescent stage the students are experiencing makes them act silly at times, thereby interrupting the session. The misinformation they have been exposed to persuades them to reject all other information initially, especially since the misinformation has originated from persons significant to them, e.g. mothers, favourite aunts or neighbours, older sisters. Owing to this, a certain amount of repetition will be needed, and this guides the second planning stage. The school authorities have decided they can give only two sessions to this health teaching. Therefore, there is only one session left.

Second session: 28 February 2003

In the first session, since I had not met the students before, I had worked on the learning need the registration teacher had identified, namely a lack of correct knowledge about menstruation. The opportunity to explore attitudes helped to generate discussion and ease the atmosphere of slight embarrassment. In the second session, I planned first to find out how much of the factual basis they remembered from the first session, and then to elicit their learning needs as they defined them and to plan the last part of the session around their needs. Therefore, the learning deficits and related needs could not be set down prior to the session.

Objectives: By the end of the second session each student will be able to:

	Learning level	Teaching strategies
1. Review the anatomy and physiology of the menstrual cycle as presented 21/2/03	Cognitive: knowledge	Oral quiz, using diagrams on overhead projector
2. List the areas related to menstruation about which she wants to know more	Cognitive: knowledge, comprehension	Brainstorm for list Put student interest list on board to decide on topics (see Box 8.3)
3. Participate in group discussions on the topics chosen	Affective: valuing	Students to break into small groups to discuss specific topic

Progress notes

The second session went well. The factual review demonstrated that most had learned the anatomy and physiology of the menstrual cycle. The problem area had to do with the hormonal changes. This was reinforced by going over the diagrams and memory device again. The brainstorming exercise pinpointed three areas of common concern: dysmenorrhoea, feminine hygiene including toxic shock syndrome, and premenstrual tension. Each area was discussed first by me. As an example, for dysmenorrhoea the following content was given:

Dysmenorrhoea or painful menstruation:

- A common problem
- Symptoms: pain, headaches, nausea, dizziness, backache, leg pain, faintness
- Two kinds:
  - primary: in the absence of pelvic disease
  - secondary: in the presence of conditions such as endometriosis
- Causes: many theories have been put forward, e.g. endocrine or hormonal imbalances, abnormal reproductive anatomy, psychogenic factors, prostaglandins
- Treatment:
  - pharmacological: use of analgesics, hormones
  - non-pharmacological: nutrition is important, decrease sodium intake, use natural diuretics to reduce fluid retention, exercise for muscle toning, mild heat, sleep and rest.

Students then met in small groups to compare notes on what they knew and how they coped (if menstruating) or have seen others cope (mothers, sisters, other female relatives or friends).

The discussion in this second session appeared to be much more serious, with little laughing and giggling. Working with the students' self-identified needs increased their motivation and participation levels. Several students expressed interest in further meetings outside of school hours. This was arranged and all were invited to attend and bring friends and mothers if desired.

EXAMPLE 3: PREOPERATIVE PREPARATION

Ward 10 is a busy gynaecological ward with a rapid turnover of patients, the vast majority of whom are in hospital for three days or less. In response to this, a fairly routinized approach to preoperative preparation has been developed. Clearly, this has disadvantages in individual cases, but the staff are convinced that the introduction of a systematic approach has been beneficial to both patients and staff. There has been no formal evaluation, since it has proved beyond their resources (both time and perhaps expertise) to design adequate outcome measures.

A previously successful venture in patient education had been the development of written sheets giving information to patients about their self-care on discharge from hospital. These were prepared jointly by the nursing and medical staff. Devising a systematic approach to preoperative care seemed the next logical step in the development of nursing practice. The medical staff had no objections, and indeed welcomed the proposals.

Assessment

It was decided that since large numbers of women pass through the ward each year, undergoing a limited range of surgical operations, it would be relatively simple to produce a list of anticipated basic information needs in relation to each type of operation. In the event, the nursing staff have been able to categorize and group certain surgical operations, because patients have very similar experiences and information needs. This case study describes the work done in relation to preparing patients to undergo laparoscopy for sterilization purposes. Although this procedure is routinely performed as a day surgery procedure and patients utilise the facilities of the day surgery unit, those who come from rural areas or the islands will have a short stay episode in the inpatient ward. Box 8.4 shows the check list of anticipated needs which was agreed by nursing and medical staff. It was decided that the nurse who prepared the patient for theatre should spend 5-10 minutes discussing these items with every patient. Since then this has been split into two short sessions, as is shown on the teaching plan which follows.

Staff were also aware of the dangers of taking a standard approach to the individual, and so it was decided that there would be some attempt to assess individual needs on admission. This is done by allowing a few minutes for discussion of the forthcoming surgery, and by recording the woman's questions and comments. These are taken as indicators of possible aids or barriers to learning, and an attempt is made to note the specific issues of concern to the patient. The assessment data are summarized. Box 8.5 shows the summary sheet for a 32-year-old legal secretary (Mrs Jones) admitted for laparoscopy.

| BOX 8.4 | *Check list of preoperative teaching needs* |

Ward 10 Preoperative information (sterilization)

Diagnosis – Check known and understood

Treatment

1. Doctor will carry out a general physical examination the evening before surgery
2. Patient must have signed consent for surgery
3. Nothing must be taken by mouth for six hours prior to surgery
4. Bathing is required in the morning before going to theatre
5. A premedication is given before theatre for inpatients (Not done for day surgery)
6. The nurse who gives the premedication will (as necessary) remove dentures, contact lenses and hair grips, and tape rings to fingers
7. There will be two small abdominal incisions closed with absorbable sutures

Progress/self-care

8. The patient will 'come round' in the recovery room
9. A cup of tea and some toast will be given once the patient is awake
10. There may be shoulder pain postoperatively because of gas used to distend the abdominal cavity to allow the surgeon to view the reproductive organs with a tele-scope-like instrument
11. The patient should stay off work for two days following discharge

Ward layout & routine

12. Location of television room
13. Smoking not permitted within hospital premises
14. Valuables have to be locked away

Learning needs

Generally, these are assumed to be the 15 information items (Box 8.4) but special note is made of individual differences, such as in Mrs Jones' case:

- the expressed fear of pain
- the expressed desire to smoke.

Planning

Because there are large numbers of patients requiring preoperative preparation for very similar operations each week, individual objectives are not always written. In all instances, there is the expectation that patients:

- must be able to recall items 3 and 13
- should be able to recall other information about treatment and preoperative care.

In Mrs Jones' case there would be further objectives related to fear of pain and smoking.

BOX 8.5	*Summary of assessment data*

Name: *Mrs Jean Jones*   Age: *32 years*

Diagnosis: *Laparoscopy for sterilization purposes*

Personal data: *stable marriage, two children, works as a legal secretary.*

Patient's questions/comments

How long will I be off work?

Can I smoke in here?

I'm an awful coward about pain.

Anticipated needs (research based)

Diagnosis

Treatment

Investigations

Prognosis ————————————— See prepared check list.

Progress

Self-care

Routine

Aids/barriers to learning

Age

Cognitive state

Educational level

Emotional level ....*Some apprehension, but otherwise no difficulties anticipated*

Grasp of technical language .....*15 items of information, but reasonably straightforward*

Hearing

Comfort

Previous experience

Sex

Motivation to learn

Attitude

Learning ability

Teaching plan

This would be detailed in the nursing notes as follows:

Timing	Staff member	Objectives	Method	Outcome
Thurs. p.m., after anaesthetist's visit	S/N Harris	1, 2	Discussion – categorize and order information items	
Wed. a.m., prior to discharge	S/N Smith	1, item 13	Discussion – elicit evidence of understanding	

The teaching task is considered to be straightforward, and the plan specifies the formal involvement of only two members of staff, though it is recognized that individual patients may ask questions of any staff member at any time, and they are encouraged to do so. The two specified nurses will fill in the outcome sections of the plan as their part in the teaching is completed. It is also made clear that there is time set aside for patients to ask questions and that both an anaesthetist and a nurse will be coming to discuss the operation with the patient prior to surgery.

Implementation

It is generally assumed that most people have at least some fears and worries about surgery, and the preoperative teaching session is geared to allaying anxiety as well as to imparting information. Attempts are made to ensure that the session, which usually lasts only five or ten minutes, will be uninterrupted and is as private as possible.

There is no guaranteed formula for success. Perhaps the most important single concern for the nurse is to attempt to listen carefully to what the woman has to say, and to avoid assuming knowledge of her thoughts and feelings. A useful approach might be to begin the discussion as follows:

'I'm Staff Nurse Harris and I'm here to talk with you about going to theatre tomorrow. I'll be telling you one or two things you will need to remember, but first tell me how you are feeling about it.' This open-ended approach may help Mrs Jones to express fears and worries. If it doesn't – for instance, if she just says, 'I'm OK' – then it is a matter of judgement as to whether it is helpful to probe further at this stage. Sometimes it helps to accept such a reply at face value and to proceed to give the information items as planned. The very act of being willing to provide information, as well as the information itself, may allay anxiety. In some instances it may be helpful to make reference to the individual's expressed concerns. In Mrs Jones' case, for instance, the fear of pain might be explored.

To assist recall, it may be useful to order and categorize information items. The essential items 3 and 13 would usually be given first. A simple categorization for other items might be 'things that happen before you go to theatre' and 'things that happen after you have had the operation'.

Evaluation

There is no formal attempt at ascertaining outcomes in terms of patients' increased satisfaction with information or of lessened anxiety, because of the measurement difficulties posed. In any case, previous research (Hayward 1975; Boore 1978; Shrestha & Poulos 2001) appears to have established that such benefits do occur. The nursing notes include a column in which staff members record subjective impressions of the outcome of teaching and note any unusual aspects of the communication process.

The examples presented in this chapter were developed to illustrate how, in the implementation phase, assessment, planning and evaluation are on-going processes which can redirect the focus of the health teacher and learner. Figure 8.2 shows where implementation fits in the teaching-learning process.

FIGURE 8.2   *The implementation process*

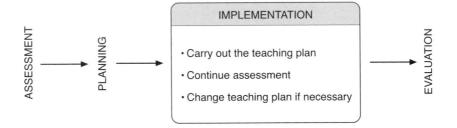

ACTIVITY 8.2

N.B. You should discuss this activity with your practice placement supervisor, tutor or mentor before you undertake it. You may need his or her advice or support during the process of carrying out the activity.

Use your initiative in the practice placement you are attached to, and identify a health teaching opportunity. If you are currently placed in a clinical area, this will probably be with an individual patient. If you are in a community placement, it might be with an individual adult or child, or it might be with a small group or a family. This will, of course depend on the specific type of placement you are in.

When you select a topic for teaching, be sure it is something that is within your present level of knowledge and skill. In any case, when you are first teaching, it is a good idea to undertake something small and easily defined. After all, as a beginning 'teacher for health', you are a learner, too. Once you have had success with small episodes of planned teaching, you can move on to more complex things.

Remember that the learning needs of your potential learner(s) must be part of the process of selecting your teaching topic. You should pick something you fancy trying to teach, but it must also be something that suits the needs of the learner. Refer to Chapter 6 as you do your needs assessment, and make notes accordingly.

Once you have carried out the needs assessment, identified and prioritised the learning needs, and selected a topic that is within the scope of your ability, you may begin planning. Refer to Chapter 7 to remind you of the elements of the planning process. Once again, make notes on your planning.

When you are satisfied with your assessment and planning, you should be ready to implement your plan. You should have gained a bit of confidence by carrying out the teaching session you did with your 'volunteer' during Activity 8.1. Now you are trying out your budding teaching skills 'for real'. As before, make notes on your teaching session, and once again, keep your notes for later use.

REFERENCES

Boore JRP 1978 Prescription for recovery. Royal College of Nursing, London.

Ewing G 1984 A study of the postoperative nursing care of stoma patients during appliance changes. Unpublished doctoral dissertation, University of Edinburgh.

Hayward J 1975 Information: a prescription against pain. Royal College of Nursing, London.

Shrestha S, Poulos A 2001 The effect of verbal information on the experience of discomfort in mammography. Radiography 7(4): 271-7.

9 Evaluating health teaching

Evaluation is an essential and inevitable part of the teaching–learning process. Whether or not the teacher plans for it to happen, both learner and teacher will evaluate, whether formally or informally. The learner may say, 'That was helpful,' or 'That was nonsense,' or 'I see what she means, but ...'. These are all evaluative statements. The teacher may say 'I did that well', or 'I made that very complicated,' or 'I explained that quite well, except for ...'. Again, these are evaluative statements.

Such informal and subjective evaluation can be useful, but it has obvious limitations. Both teacher and learner need more detailed and constructive feedback. The teacher should not be content with an intuitive sense that all went well, but should attempt to identify exactly what has been achieved. There are two reasons for this: to provide guidance as to how to improve one's teaching; and to contribute to the needs assessment for further teaching. Likewise, the learner should aim to assess his or her grasp of new knowledge, or acceptance of the ideas proposed.

In a constructive teaching and learning environment, where intuitive assessment is enhanced by a planned approach, both teacher and learner may have to develop the skills of planned evaluation. In some situations they may even do this jointly. For example, in cases of psychiatric illness or spinal cord injury, where rehabilitation is a complex and long-term process, both nurse and patient have much to learn together, and will develop skills in setting goals and assessing outcomes as part of that process of learning. More commonly, however, the nurse, as teacher, will assist the patient or client, as learner, to acquire the relevant skills.

THE BENEFITS OF PLANNED EVALUATION

Planned evaluation is an important part of the health teaching process for a number of reasons. Firstly, it gives tangible evidence of what has been accomplished. This motivates the learner and helps the nurse gain job satisfaction and confidence in her teaching role.

Secondly, evaluation provides the means to weigh achievement against stated goals. This allows the possibility of planned future improvements. Every teaching programme has to be adjusted to the individual learner, the talents of the teacher, and the environment in which teaching takes place. Often such adjustment is immediate, in response to learner needs within a given teaching opportunity. Such spontaneous and often intuitive adjustment may, however, be backed by a planned and documented approach to evaluation. Sometimes it is only by reflecting on the teaching process in retrospect that useful feedback can be provided. Planned evaluation exercises should incorporate the learner's views along with the teacher's, and make intuitive reactions subject to a degree of objectivity, perhaps even measurement. Pure objectivity is, of course, impossible, since the teaching–learning event is an activity involving human interaction, and whatever evaluation process is employed, it is formulated and operated by persons with subjective views. However, this does not discount the value of seeking whatever degree of objectivity is possible.

A third reason for evaluating is to provide evidence that health teaching is worthwhile, in terms of what it costs. Sometimes this is a relatively easy exercise. For instance, research has demonstrated that giving information to patients as a preparation for surgery has proved to be beneficial in reducing the amount of analgesia required and the incidence of postoperative infection (Hayward 1975; Boore 1978) and that providing information in writing and through a personal visit could change back pain behaviour (Roberts et al 2002). It is possible to calculate such benefits and thus demonstrate the *cost-effectiveness* and *cost-benefit* of health education (Naidoo & Wills 2000; Cohen & Hale 2002).

It should be noted, however, that health education and promotion, along with many other aspects of health care, cannot always be justified on economic grounds alone. Health education in the prevention of heart disease provides a good example of this problem, since it can be argued that it might be cheaper to let people die of coronary artery disease than to sustain the costs of care in old age. It can also be argued that there are benefits other than economic ones that are at least equally important, so it follows that cost benefit alone does not amount to sufficient grounds for judging the value of a health education activity.

The cost equation itself is very complicated. How are costs of lost production to be estimated? Or the costs of a teenager losing a father? Besides, health educators might argue (though research evidence on this needs strengthening) that health education can contribute to a fitter and more independent old age, thus reducing costs of caring for the elderly.

Despite the difficulties, there are increasing demands, in times of financial stringency, to demonstrate the benefits of health education in financial terms, and this aspect of evaluation should be a primary concern of anyone planning for health teaching. Indeed, planners may require the individual health educator to demonstrate not only that health education makes financial sense in relation to other aspects of health care, but that the particular programme of health education recommended is *cost effective*. A cost-effective programme is one which achieves the health care objectives most efficiently; in other words, at similar or less cost than other programmes achieving comparable results.

Other reasons for carrying out evaluation reflect social and emotional as well as practical considerations. For instance, if health teaching is to mean the difference between feeling well and being very ill, as in severe diabetes mellitus, then evaluation of the extent of learning, in this case about the use of insulin, diet and energy expenditure, will be essential. At the end of the day, the issue of how health teaching benefits the recipient may be as important as the consideration of costs. Being pain-free in the postoperative stage sooner than the average patient is likely to be more important to the patient than is any reduction in the cost of analgesia. Considering the subjective view of the individual is also important in relation to research findings. In a study of the effects of information and support on individuals awaiting cadaveric kidney transplantation, Russell and Brown (2002) found no statistical evidence for the effectiveness of the intervention, according to the quantitative outcome measures they used. However, participants in the study indicated that they felt definite needs had been met for them by the information and support intervention. Thus evaluation of the usefulness of health education should be geared to the recipient's as well as the planner's or researcher's view of utility.

The nurse who evaluates his or her health teaching demonstrates a willingness to be held accountable for it. He or she is able to show, through judgement which may incorporate measurement, whether or not his or her efforts were effective. If learning has not occurred, evaluation helps to pinpoint reasons and provides the basis of re-assessment from which further planning, teaching and evaluation may proceed.

A caveat should be added here, and that is that a direct and exclusive cause-and-effect relationship cannot often safely be assumed to exist between the teaching and the learning. The teacher is not the only influence on how effectively an intended learner learns. This is true for both positive and negative results. If the learner does not learn, it is not necessarily the fault of the teaching, and if the learner does learn, it is not necessarily because (certainly not only because) of the teaching. This does not imply that there is therefore no real point in evaluating; instead it implies that one of the elements that should be evaluated, if possible, is the extent to which it was the teaching that made the difference. It further implies the importance of evaluating the other factors that influenced the learning.

DEFINING EVALUATION

Evaluation, then, is a planned process and should be continuous; it is made in regard to stated criteria, which may be developed and applied by both teacher and learner, and may involve measurement. The steps in evaluation are:

1. Consider the objectives of the health teaching.
2. Identify the object of interest for the evaluation: knowledge, attitudes or behaviour.

3. Design the evaluation programme.
4. Select or devise measurements.
5. Collect and analyse data.
6. Record the results and provide feedback.

Educationalists (Bloom et al 1971; Guilbert 1977; Bastable 2003) distinguish between *formative* and *summative* evaluation. The term 'formative' is applied to evaluation used as a continuous process which provides feedback throughout the teaching and learning event. This type of evaluation helps to determine the pace and extent of learning and allows the health teacher to vary teaching activity to meet the learner's needs. Formative evaluation is a mechanism which enhances the teaching–learning situation. In this way it is different from the 'summative' evaluation which is done at the end of a teaching–learning programme specifically to identify how much has been learned. Most people have experienced summative evaluation in the form of final school exams which determine whether or not one progresses to another educational level, or what level of educational award is to be given, and it may be for this reason that evaluation is often assumed to be concerned only with end results. However, both types of evaluation are necessary in health teaching, and in this text the distinction between types of evaluation is further refined by use of three terms which are used fairly commonly in health care evaluation. These are: structure, process and outcome.

AREAS OF EVALUATION: STRUCTURE, PROCESS, OUTCOME

Structure, process and outcome are three areas of evaluation which help to analyse the who, what and how of the health education process (see Figure 9.1). Comprehensive evaluation will encompass all three areas.

| FIGURE 9.1 | *Comprehensive evaluation includes consideration of structure, process and outcome measures* |

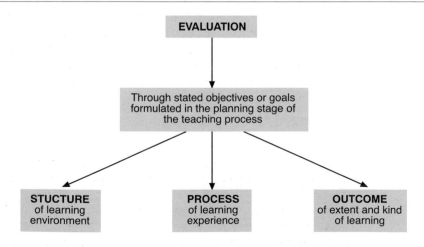

BOX 9.1	*Evaluation of structure – some guiding questions*

- What topics were dealt with?
- Which staff were involved?
- Were the facilities and resources adequate?
- Was there enough time?
- Was the environment conducive to learning?
- Were the mechanisms for judging learner satisfaction adequate?

Structure

Evaluation of structure is concerned with aspects of the learning environment, including the availability and use of such factors as premises, expertise, equipment and human resources. Structural evaluation is characterized by consideration of the availability and accessibility of teaching and looks at what was organized for teaching. In a hospital setting the concern might be with the success of the provision of privacy or timing of post-discharge instructions. In the community, structural evaluation might aim at determining whether the location of the clinic where classes were held was influential in encouraging people to attend or whether the supply of audiovisual equipment gave ease of access to all. In the home, it might consider the degree of comfort of the surroundings and the level of distractions. Additionally, structural evaluation relates to such elements as records of topics covered and numbers attending, and means used for monitoring the satisfaction of learners.

This type of evaluation is necessary to good planning, but it has limitations. It is not enough to know that there was a good turnout at a health education film or that most people seemed satisfied. Equally, information about the proportion of patients who received preoperative instruction and which members of staff were involved, is of little use in the absence of any evidence of the success of such instruction. On the other hand, negative evaluation of facilities, resources or surroundings may exist along with a positive evaluation of the results of the teaching. In other words, a positive evaluation of the structure will not make up for a lack of learning, nor will a negative evaluation of the structure discount a good learning result. Some excellent teaching and learning can take place under difficult circumstances, and ideal circumstances do not guarantee good teaching and learning. Box 9.1 suggests a set of questions to guide the evaluation of structure.

Process

Evaluation of process deals with how resources were used, which types of technique were employed, and how appropriate these resources and techniques were in relation to the particular learner(s) and the learning task in hand. Such evaluation is a joint venture between the health teacher and the learner(s).

In part, what is being analysed is the art of teaching. What took place? How was it organized? This is the act of relating the subject matter and the objec-

| BOX 9.2 | *Evaluation of process – some guiding questions* |

The learner

■ Were the learner's perceptions of his need for health teaching elicited?

■ Was the learner involved in the selection of learning method?

■ How did the learner participate?

■ Were there fluctuations in the level of participation?

■ What kind of responses did the learner make?

The health teacher

■ Was the teacher credible to the learners?

■ Which teaching style was used, and was it appropriate?

■ Was the teacher's performance organized?

■ Did the teacher relate positively to the learners?

■ Was the interaction active and was discussion allowed?

■ Did the teacher listen to the learners?

■ Was the teacher consistent, accepting and respectful towards the learners?

■ Did the teacher provide feedback?

■ Did the teacher appear knowledgeable?

The method and aids

■ What methods were used?

■ Were the methods learner-centred or teacher-centred?

■ Did these methods build on experience and ability?

■ Were the learners motivated and stimulated by the methods?

■ What aids were used?

■ Did the aids contribute positively to the presentation?

■ Were the aids visible/audible to the learner(s)?

■ Did the teacher handle the aids well?

The content

■ Was the content logically organized?

■ Was the amount right, both for the capacity of the learners and for the allotted time?

■ Did the content relate to and build upon the learner's previous knowledge and experience?

The objectives or goals

■ Was the choice of the objectives or other approach suitable to the teaching task?

■ Were the objectives specific, realistic and meaningful in relation to the health education needs of the individual?

■ Were the objectives appropriately worded?

■ If a non-objectives approach was used, was it effective for the purpose?

■ Were the learners aware of the objectives or goals?

tives to a series of tasks and activities. The term 'process' refers to what happens between teacher and learner. Setting out to help a person to learn how to administer an injection involves visualizing the end result, and planning the teaching in stages which will achieve that result. The likely approach is to use demonstration or a videotape to show the technique of injection, then break the skill into a set of subroutines. At each point, various methods and techniques are available to reinforce learning and to evaluate progress so far. Choice of these, along with everything else that occurs, may help or hinder the learning experience. Thus the process of learning and teaching should be recorded fully to allow examination of positive and negative influences on learning. A process recording technique is discussed later in this chapter, and an example is shown in Box 9.10 (page 205).

The essence of good process evaluation is to provide for constructive feedback, both throughout the learning and at the end. Without the facility for feedback throughout, learning may proceed slowly and inefficiently. The learner will experience a certain amount of intrinsic feedback in the act of learning. However, his own self-assessment is seldom enough, and constructive comment from the health teacher is essential to motivation. In some instances it may be necessary to help the learner identify and acknowledge his attainments. Learners are often more conscious of and ready to acknowledge their shortcomings than their strengths. The quality of the assessment and the way it is given are important considerations: feedback should be informative, reinforcing and motivating. To achieve these three requirements, it may also need to be tactful.

Box 9.2 contains sets of questions that can guide the evaluation of process.

Outcome

Evaluation of outcome is concerned with end results. For this, some kind of measurement is usually required. The desired outcomes of health teaching may be defined as changes in knowledge, attitudes and/or behaviour. A necessary first step in evaluation is the clarification of the purpose of the health education programme, in order to identify suitable outcome measures. If the programme seeks to influence behaviour, then measures of changed knowledge or attitude will not suffice, since it can be demonstrated that the link between knowledge or attitudes and behaviour is uncertain. At the same time, it is unrealistic, and unfair, to apply measures of behavioural outcome to a programme designed only to achieve knowledge or awareness.

Evaluating affective learning

Measurements of attitude change are difficult both to construct and to apply. For this reason, and because there is doubt about the link between attitudes and behaviour, measures of health teaching outcome are commonly sought in relation to knowledge factors or to behaviour. It is possible, however, to address attitudes in a non-scientific way by providing opportunities for the learner to talk about the topic and express his views, after the learning event. This can be done to a certain extent towards the end of a teaching session, or the end of a series of sessions. True attitude change cannot be assumed from immediate expression, however, so in a situation where the health teacher has ongoing contact with the learner, views elicited over time may be more telling.

Evaluating cognitive learning

Instruments to measure knowledge are fairly easily constructed but may be difficult to apply. The knowledge review that follows Chapter 11 in this book provides an example of such an instrument. Although it does contain items related to affective and psychomotor aspects of learning, their effectiveness for this purpose is severely limited. The case for psychological manipulation, for example, and the value of health education, both affective issues, are addressed, but the answers elicited might or might not represent the genuine views of the student writing them. The student might express what he or she considers to be the correct or acceptable point of view rather than the view he or she actually holds. In addition, such questions by the very nature of their content do not have correct answers. In the psychomotor realm, the use of audiovisual aids and the assessment of a new baby are indirectly addressed, but the answers to those items would not provide evidence of mastery of the psychomotor skills involved. In contrast, most of the questions in the review represent a check on cognitive learning, and the answers to these will demonstrate the level of knowledge acquired and can be assessed for correctness.

Students expect this sort of evaluation or examination of their learning to take place. Adults, however, whether in hospital, attending a family planning clinic, a series of prenatal classes or a single lecture on the causes of alcoholism, may find knowledge questionnaires threatening or even insulting. As with affective learning, it may be possible to do some evaluation of cognitive learning towards the end of a learning episode by eliciting feedback from the learner about the material that has been covered. However, the same problem also holds true: the immediate evidence cannot be assumed to represent true learning. Once again, if possible, if there is longer-term contact between the health teacher and the learner, later evidence of learning may be obtained.

Evaluating psychomotor learning

The measurement of behaviour presents a considerable challenge, because behavioural outcomes vary in the extent to which they are observable and amenable to reliable recording. In relation to activities which entail the teaching of specific skills to individuals or small groups, many types of psychomotor learning can be readily observed. The patient who has been taught to test her urine and blood, calculate her insulin dosage and administer it by injection can be observed carrying out these behaviours. This can be done in stages as the learning is taking place, and it can be done summatively once the teaching–learning activities are complete. In addition, it can be checked again on subsequent occasions over time. Some other examples of psychomotor learning are less readily observed and evaluated. It is quite simple, for instance, to demonstrate the correct way to apply a condom, and to get a return demonstration from the learner. These will be done in contrived circumstances, however, using inanimate aids. It is virtually impossible (and usually inappropriate) to observe the learner actually applying a condom in real life.

In relation to both the examples mentioned above – the insulin injection and the condom application – there is an additional confounding factor. That is that the performance of the learned behaviours does not depend solely on the psychomotor learning. A person may know how to test blood and urine, and

BOX 9.3	*Some health indicators*

Vital statistics	*Health behaviour statistics*
Birth rate	Use of services
Mortality	Preventive actions
Population growth	Consumption patterns
Social statistics	*Disease statistics*
Illegitimacy	Morbidity
Unemployment	Disability
Absenteeism	Restriction to activity

know how to calculate the dosage and administer the insulin, but that does not ensure that he or she will do it. Similarly, a person may be perfectly able to apply a condom correctly, and yet the person or the person's partner may fail to use one at the appropriate time. Thus it is not the learning of technical skills alone that keeps diabetes in control, or prevents unwanted pregnancy or the transmission of HIV. Clearly the accompanying cognitive learning is critical to the subsequent correct performance of the psychomotor learning, but the relevant affective learning is perhaps even more instrumental in determining whether the learned behaviour will be carried out. Thus the evaluation of psychomotor learning, which at first glance appears to be relatively straightforward, can be exceedingly complex.

Evaluation at the community level

In addition to the perspective of the individual or small group teaching–learning activity, wider evidence of such learning is often sought. Box 9.3 shows some of the indicators that may be used (see also Chapter 1). Some behavioural outcomes may be observed, recorded and measured readily on a population-wide basis. The use of a specific service such as chiropody or dental services is an example. Vital indicators, such as morbidity, mortality and fertility, are also readily available, though negative, health indices. Others, such as preventive actions, consumption patterns or rates of compliance with prescribed drug regimens, are less easily observed. In such cases, recording may depend on self-reports and clearly these are subject to bias. Some indicators such as teenage pregnancy, unemployment and absenteeism are easily recorded but less easily interpreted in health terms. There have been attempts at producing reliable health indices which will reflect social, emotional and physical functioning (Culyer 1983), but there is still some way to go before indices are developed which will satisfy the needs of health care planners and fully reflect experiences and views of health seen as relevant by members of the public.

A further point that is worth considering in relation to outcomes of health teaching is that there can be outcomes that relate more to the process itself than to the subject matter. These may be intentional goals or unintentional by-products. They include what are sometimes referred to as personal transferable skills – skills such as the ability to discuss, explain, persuade, negotiate, tolerate, compromise, argue constructively, and so on. One very important such outcome, especially in health education within the community, is the empowerment of the individual. This entails the acquisition of self-confidence and assertiveness skills, the ability to make considered decisions and to assert control over one's own life and health within the social system in which one lives.

SETTING EVALUATION CRITERIA

If the purpose of evaluation is to weigh achievement against aims, then it is necessary to establish criteria for judging success. In individualized health teaching, when an objectives-based approach has been used, the instructional objectives, properly written, will specify these, and this can be done in negotiation with the patient. In health teaching using a non-objectives-based approach, and in community-based programmes, however, it may be more difficult to establish what change in knowledge or behaviour constitutes success.

The use of standards

Somehow, a standard has to be set. Green (1974) looked at a number of studies and identified different standards of acceptability for patient education outcomes. One of these was the *absolute standard* wherein the standard is set by policy-makers who have opted for an unrealistic 100% solution. An example of this might be to expect a series of sessions with a group of smokers to result in all participants becoming permanent non-smokers. This is not a reasonable expectation, either for the teacher or for the participants.

Equally unsatisfactory, at the other extreme, is the *arbitrary standard*, based upon whim or hunch. Here the example might be represented by an expectation that, to be considered successful, the series of sessions should encourage the members to stop smoking. Such a standard is vague, and it leaves open the question of what 'being encouraged' means.

Sometimes it is possible to establish a *historical standard*, by looking at trends relating to the individual's personal history, the population at risk or the health problem. This might be expressed as a statement indicating that as a result of the health teaching sessions, the participants should, on average, have decreased their smoking by at least 30% as compared with the amount they smoked before. Their rate of smoking after the health teaching is thus measured against their rate of smoking before, and success is judged accordingly.

The use of *normative standards* involves comparison with the outcomes of programmes carried out for similar reasons, with like populations in similar environments. An example in this case might be that the stop-smoking sessions should result in a proportion of the participants becoming non-smokers in line with the degree of success in a similar programme in an EU country that has achieved a meaningful decrease in smoking behaviour. This provides a sounder basis for standard setting, though it is not foolproof. If rates of smoking are decreasing in all EU countries, then achieving a rate that appears to be behind the rest might still be a significant improvement. On the other hand, if rates

| BOX 9.4 | *Evaluation of outcome – some guiding questions* |

The learner

- What were the changes in knowledge and/or behaviour?
- Can any inferences be drawn as to changes in attitudes, values or beliefs?
- Was there any evidence of an increased ability to analyse, to participate, to adapt health actions?
- Was there evidence of transferable skills or empowerment being gained?
- Did the learner consider he or she benefited?

The health teacher

- Did the teacher's health knowledge or behaviour change?
- Were insights into health-related behaviour gained?
- Was the teacher able to reflect on his or her own performance in order to improve his or her teaching skills?

The method and aids

- Did the method used achieve the desired results?
- Was it more economical than other comparable methods?
- Would other methods have been more appropriate?
- Were any aids used effective for the purpose?

The objectives

- Were they achievable?
- Were they measurable? By which standards?
- Were they met?
- Whose objectives or goals were met?
- If intended goals or objectives were not achieved, why not?

are high in all EU countries, then even being better than all the rest would not necessarily mean a high achievement, in a real sense.

The use of *theoretical standards*, or those based on predictions from theory or on previous research, is another potentially sound standard. In this case, the success of the stop-smoking programme would be judged according to a standard which has been found to be both possible and health-promoting, on the basis of careful scrutiny of the literature from the biological and behavioural sciences on the subject.

Sometimes a *negotiated standard* can be set in which the desired change in behaviour is jointly determined, as can happen in care managed on the basis of a contract between professionals and clients. In the example here, this would imply a contract agreed between the group and the health teacher, between individual participants and the health teacher, or among the members of the whole group, as to what amount of decrease in smoking activity would count as success.

Box 9.4 offers some questions that can be used to guide the evaluation of outcome.

EVALUATION DESIGNS FOR OUTCOME ASSESSMENT

One of the challenges of recording the outcomes of health teaching is to find adequate and positive indices of health. In addition, even where acceptable and reliable outcome measures exist, it may be difficult to establish that any change in health-related knowledge or behaviour can be attributed to the particular health teaching intervention. Careful choice of an experimental or quasi-experimental research design may help.

Consider four common evaluation designs, shown in Box 9.5. In Design 1 the only observations or measurements occurred after the health teaching. Therefore, the evaluation cannot determine whether or not there has been any change in the learner's knowledge level or health behaviour.

Design 2, because it includes a pre-test, is more useful, but there are limitations. It does not allow for changes which might have occurred over time in any case: subjects may have matured, or they may have been influenced by another educational experience such as a television programme. It is also possible that the pre-test influenced the post-test, by sensitizing the learner to the focus of the teaching–learning event. This is less of a concern in health teaching than it would be in pure research, since pre-testing is often part of the teaching strategy and may be used to motivate learners.

Design 3 uses the concept of control as a way around some of the problems found in the pre- and post-test design. Use of control groups can help isolate the effects of the health teaching intervention. This design requires that the experimental group is taught and tested. The control group is tested at the same point(s) but is not taught. This offers some improvement as a method, but again there are limitations because the pre-test does not establish the detailed characteristics of the groups. It has to be assumed that they are comparable.

In pure research this problem can be minimized by careful choice of control and statistical application with sufficiently large samples. In health education, however, this presents problems in practice because it may mean using a questionnaire type of evaluation with possible resulting superficiality of data. It may also mean that the health teaching to be applied is equally superficial, in order to achieve adequately sized samples. The research phenomenon, that it is possible to achieve either a large representative sample with superficial data or a data-rich study carried out in a sample which is either small or has no adequate control group, presents a particular challenge to the health educator (Green 1977).

Design 4 offers one possible solution to the problem of finding a research design that will demonstrate conclusively the effects of any teaching intervention. The answer lies in using randomly allocated learners. This fourth design is similar to the third one, but the random allocation of subjects into groups means that initial differences in the two groups are equalized by randomization. In terms of the research problem this is a neat solution. For the health educator, however, some difficulties remain. There is often still a problem of inadequate numbers to make any findings statistically significant. When findings are not statistically significant, no real weight can be given to any differences that are found, because they may be attributable to mere coincidence. In other words, the random allocation within small numbers cannot ensure equalization of characteristics across the groups.

BOX 9.5	Four evaluation designs

Key: O = observation*   R = random allocation   X = teaching

1. Post-test only	All participants		X	O
2. Pre- and post-test	All participants	O_1	X	O_2
3. Using a control group	Experimental group	O_1	X	O_2
	Control group	O_1		O_2
4. Random allocation of	Experimental group	R	X	O
persons into groups	Control group	R		O

* 'Observation' may take various forms, e.g. written test, visual observation with check list, oral account of individual perceptions.

Another problem is that it may be difficult to achieve random allocation of people into groups. This is particularly the case in community education where groups are often self-selecting. This design can, however, be applied where groups are convened by health educators themselves (such as for prenatal classes) who thus have control over the flow of members. It may also be applicable in patient education, provided any ethical issues about the withholding of information can be resolved. If too much information about the evaluation study is given to the learners, that knowledge may influence the way they behave. If too little information is given, the procedure may be thought to be unethical, in that informed consent was not given by the participants.

Techniques of evaluation: issues of validity and reliability

Techniques of evaluation help to gather information which, when interpreted, assesses if and how learning has occurred. As has been stressed, the techniques must be designed to measure the kind or kinds of learning specified in the objectives or goals for the educational programme. Two qualities of measurement are additional essential considerations: validity and reliability.

When a method or technique of measurement is valid, it has measured what it was intended to measure. For instance, assessing the effects of senior citizens' exercise programmes on flexibility of movement by giving a written questionnaire would be an invalid method. Observing exercises in progress or actually measuring how much the senior citizens can flex and extend limbs would be a valid approach.

The second term, reliability, refers to the consistency of a measurement tool. If a health visitor, concerned with the incidence of ischaemic heart disease in the community, tested the knowledge level of her clients about the health risks of smoking, the results should be the same on one day as on the next. That is, the tool should generate consistent responses provided there has been no intervening teaching or experience to change the responders' knowledge. In addition, to be reliable, the tool should give results which agree with other valid tests of the same knowledge, if such tests exist.

A wide range of evaluation techniques is available. Figure 9.2 indicates how they might be applied in the evaluation of structure, process and outcome. Not all techniques are practical for everyday health teaching; the nurse or midwife will need to judge which is appropriate and feasible for a given instance of teaching.

Oral questioning

This is a readily available, and thus valuable, tool for the health teacher, for in most nursing situations the evaluation of learning may need to be immediate and ongoing. Questioning is a central critical element in health teaching because it promotes thinking about the subject under discussion. In evaluation, questioning permits the health teacher to check comprehension, to test knowledge, and to diagnose weaknesses in the learner's knowledge base. It also offers an opportunity to make some assessment of attitudes, values and beliefs.

How the questions are posed is important. Chapter 4 reviewed therapeutic communication and provided guidelines about formulating questions. It is important to remember that the value of oral questioning as an evaluation technique will be enhanced in many instances if answers are recorded.

Questionnaire surveys

These have a useful but limited application in relation to evaluation of structural factors and learner satisfaction. Good survey forms often look deceptively simple, but achieving validity and reliability can be difficult. Each question should be carefully considered and pilot-tested. Useful further reading sources on this and the other techniques in this section are noted at the end of this chapter.

Check lists

These are quite commonly used in patient education, usually as a reminder of content to be included. They also have a role to play in evaluation. Boxes 9.6 and 9.7 show two check lists. The first might be used in process evaluation, to check the content of preoperative teaching. The second could be applied as an outcome measure to indicate whether someone with a newly formed colostomy has grasped the sequence involved in an appliance change. This check list provides a reminder of the sequence and evidence that the learner is following it, except for inspecting the skin area and providing skin care. This would be a point for discussion. The check list is useful as far is it goes, but it does not address the level or quality of learning achieved, merely the coverage of items.

Rating scales

These have their origins in psychological research. Traditionally they were used to assess attitudes. A typical rating scale consists of a list of statements of opinion, against which people indicate their level of agreement in such terms as 'strongly agree', 'agree', 'disagree', 'strongly disagree'. Rating scales may be widely applied in the evaluation of health teaching. They can be completed by the learner, to give the teacher a view of the learner's knowledge or views, or they can be completed by the teacher about the learner. In the former case, the

FIGURE 9.2   *Evaluation techniques used to assess the structure, process and outcome of the teaching–learning situation*

Evaluation area	Oral questioning	Questionnaire survey	Check list	Rating scale	Written tests	Diaries	Process recording	Nursing audit
I STRUCTURE								
1. Facilities, resources, time allocation	x	x	x	x				x
2. Learning aids	x	x	x	x				x
II PROCESS								
1. Participation and response of learner	x		x	x		x	x	
2. Health teacher characteristics			x	x		x		
3. Effectiveness of method used	x		x	x				x
4. Content organization			x	x				x
III OUTCOME								
1. Learning accomplished	x			x	x	x		
2. Teacher insight increased			x	x		x		
3. Goal and objective achievement				x	x	x		x
4. Programme value				x		x		x

learner might rate a statement such as 'Smoking makes me feel relaxed' or 'I feel that the sessions were well organized' according to the categories mentioned above. With respect to the latter case, Box 9.8 shows how a rating scale item might be constructed to assess skill learning related to stoma care.

Written tests

These have wide application in some forms of health teaching; for instance, they may be applied within a school health education programme. In many situations, however, particularly in patient education, a written test will provide an unnecessary threat, so they should be used with care.

Some questions can help guide the construction of written tests:

- Is the material worth a test?
- Is the learner physically and emotionally able to take the test?
- Is this the best way of evaluating what has been learned?
- Is the test at the reading and comprehension level of the learner?
- Are the directions clear?
- Has unnecessary jargon been avoided?

BOX 9.6	*Check list for preoperative preparation*

Information items

Signing of operation consent	Anaesthetic room procedure
Visit from the anaesthetist	Recovery
Arrangements for fasting	Visiting
Timing of surgery	Details of anticipated surgery
Timing of premedication	Postoperative expectations:
Activity following premedication	– IV
Emptying of bladder	– drains
Removal of items:	– position
– jewellery	– food and fluids
– hair clips	– activity
– dentures	

BOX 9.7	*Stoma care appliance change check list*

Action sequence	Patient followed sequence	
	Yes	No
Chose location for change	✓	
Gathered equipment	✓	
Removed old appliance	✓	
Inspected skin area		✓
Provided skin care		✓
Measured stoma	✓	
Fitted new appliance	✓	
Tidied up	✓	

BOX 9.8	*Rating scale item*

Objective: The client inspects and describes the condition of the area of skin around the stoma with each change.

1	2	3
Did not inspect skin condition	Looked at area briefly, did not describe skin condition	Carefully examined skin area around stoma and described condition

BOX 9.9	'Objective' test items

True/False: The statements below are either true or false. Note in the space provided before each statement whether you believe it is true (T) or false (F).

_____ 1. Ischaemic heart disease is one of the most common causes of death in Britain.

_____ 2. You cannot catch HIV or AIDS by just sharing a needle once.

Fill in the blank: In each statement below a word is missing. Fill in the word you believe correctly completes the statement.

1. The factor that contributes most to the development of lung cancer is

....

2. The drop in blood sugar that occurs if there is too much insulin in the bloodstream is called

....

Matching: Below are two columns of words. From the right column select words which indicate the main type of dietary substance contained in items in the left column. Enter the letter of the right-hand column word beside the number of the left-hand column word.

_____ 1. bread   a. fat

_____ 2. poached haddock   b. protein

_____ 3. margarine   c. carbohydrate

4. pasta

_____ 5. olive oil

Multiple choice: Below are statements or questions followed by a selection of possible answers. Select the answer or answers you believe is/are correct by circling the letter or letters preceding the correct answer or answers.

1. When a diabetic person has missed a meal, a possible result might be:

   a. Ketoacidosis

   b. Hyperglycaemia

   c. Hypoglycaemia

   d. Hypertension

2. Smoking may be a factor in the cause of:

   a. Coronary artery disease

   b. Lung cancer

   c. Stroke

   d. Cancer of the urinary bladder

Box 9.9 contains examples of items that might be used to make up a written test of the 'objective' type. The term 'objective' is used in this sense to mean that the marking of such a test is objective. It is not, of course, objective in the making, since the teacher or tester subjectively decides what will be asked and what will constitute a correct answer. A particular problem with using this type of test is the danger of testing only trivial material, merely because it lends itself the most easily to testing. If this happens, then the test as a whole cannot be said to be valid, because it does not cover the information in correct balance.

Learners may also be asked to write answers to open-ended questions, similar to what students are used to as 'essay questions'. Here again, care must be used, because such testing may be anxiety-provoking for the learner, and it may bring an unnecessarily formal atmosphere into the teaching–learning situation. It may be more appropriate to explore the material with the learner orally.

Diaries

Diaries may provide useful material for evaluation. They can be used by both health teacher and learner to record personal observations about their own reactions to and feelings about a teaching–learning situation. The entries are then compared and analysed for changes in attitude and feelings and even behaviour. Learner diaries can be used to assess the reaction to the structure and process of the learning situation. Teacher diaries may provide insight for the individual health teacher as to his own feelings and reactions.

Process recordings

These can help to analyse the effectiveness of the teaching–learning process. Box 9.10 illustrates how a process recording can assist examination of the content and feeling of the interaction between the learner and health teacher. Mr Hughes does not appear to be ready to proceed with learning about colostomy care. The nurse considers whether or not her approach was a contributing factor in Mr Hughes' response.

Nursing audits

These may provide the context of health teaching evaluation, usually as part of a quality assurance programme. The function of a nursing audit is to determine the level of care given, as set against a defined standard, and to provide evidence of the success or failure of nursing care. Nursing audits may be accomplished by a single nurse, but more often a peer group or the care team will examine nursing care plans to determine the adequacy of care.

The health teaching strengths of the nursing team may be built up through the process of nursing audit. The essence of the audit is to provide time to reflect on the assumed purposes, the process and the outcome of health teaching in a given environment, be it ward, clinic, health centre, school, industrial premises or whatever. The audit operates by providing opportunities for constructive feedback. Patients, clients, and the entire care team may have a part to play in this learning process from time to time. However, on a day-to-day basis, the audit will be managed by the nursing staff, and much of the activity will centre on detailed examination of the nursing care plan. In relation to

BOX 9.10	*Illustration of a process recording*

What the patient said and did (verbal and nonverbal communication)	What the nurse said and did	Analysis
	I noticed from the chart that Mr Hughes, a patient with a recent colostomy, had not begun to learn how to care for his stoma. I decided to assess his readiness for learning. I went to his bed on the ward, introduced myself, and said, 'Mr Hughes, I see you have had a colostomy and that the nurses have been changing the appliance for you.'	This was the first time I had met Mr Hughes. Perhaps it might have been better for one of the nurses who has been caring for him to make the approach. I noted his immediate reticence but decided to proceed. I may have made him feel guilty by the way I opened the conservation.
Looked uncomfortable. Replied 'yes.' Not volunteering anything else.		
	'Do you have any questions about the colostomy?'	
'No.' Sounded angry.		
		'Tell me what's been happening with your colostomy?' or 'How do you feel you're getting on?' might have been better as a first question.

FIGURE 9.3 Teaching plan for learning about stoma appliance management showing use in evaluation *Ewing 1984*

GUIDELINES	CARE DETAILS	9/9/02	10/9	11/9	12/9	13/9	14/9
Preparation of equipment	Tray To ward bathroom	A	A	AT	G	G	SC
Preparation of patient	Location Wd brm Position Sitting Time After breakfast	A	AT	AT	G	G	SC
Removal of old appliance	Method Gentle peel	A	AT	AT	G	S	SC
Skin care	Cleanser drying agent Soap & water	A	AT	AT	AT	G	G
Skin protection	Intact ✓ Damaged Broken	A	AT	AT	AT	G	G
Selection of new appliance	Effluent—fluid ✓ firm Type Coloplast drainable Size 40	A	A	AT	G	G	SC
Preparation of appliance	Method Measure with guide cut & peel	A	A	AT	AT	G	SC
Application	Angle Vertical Accessories belt Closure Surgical clips	A	A	AT	AT	G	SC
Disposal	Method Ward toilets	A	A	AT	G	G	SC

Helping method (enter code under date)

Acting—A
Teaching—T
Guiding—G
Supporting—S
Home care/ self care—SC

Developmental & environmental reminders:

Privacy
Uninterrupted care
Exposure of stoma only
Screening of patient
Terminology
Facial expression
No gloves

Patient details

Name: Jane Smith
Date of birth: 8/3/57
Diagnosis: Cancer of the cervix
Operation: Laparotomy, colostomy

Type of stoma
ileostomy
colostomy ✓

Site of stoma
ileum
ascending colon
transverse colon
descending colon
sigmoid colon ✓

Form of stoma
end
loop ✓
double barrel

Length of stoma
spout
flush ✓
retracted

Physical condition
eyesight uses glasses
hearing good
manual deformity none
skin problems none

Home conditions:
toilet facilities—bathroom
means of disposal—city rubbish collection

COMMENTS

Works as librarian in local public library.
Lives with husband (bank manager). 1 daughter lives at home, age 20, university student. 1 married daughter lives in New York.
Allergic to penicillin.

ACTIVITY 9.1

In this activity, you will evaluate the teaching activity you carried out for Activity 8.1. You will do this in two parts.

Evaluating the teaching plan and the teaching event

Write notes on the effectiveness of the teaching by answering the following questions:

- How well did your plan work?
- Was the time adequate to accomplish the task?
- Were there points in the teaching–learning session when you had to be flexible? If so, how did you modify your teaching? Did your plan allow for this?
- Were there things you would do differently on another similar occasion?
- What were the good points about your teaching session, things you would be sure to remember for another time?

Evaluating the learning

To do this, you will need to decide what means of evaluation to use. Consider the techniques discussed in this chapter, and select one or more that you think is/are appropriate to the teaching you did. If possible, carry out the evaluation. If this is not possible, just write notes about how you would do it. In the end, try to answer the following questions:

- What was the nature of the learning that took place (cognitive, psychomotor, or affective; surface-level or deep-level, etc.)?
- To what extent were the learning goals or objectives achieved?
- What should the next health learning be for this individual?

health teaching, teaching plans can be scrutinized to identify a number of factors, such as:

- How did the plan proceed?
- To what extent did the learner achieve the objectives?
- How did the nurses record teaching sessions? Is the recording concise, informative and easily understood?

Clearly, the adequacy of documentation will be vital to the process of audit. One concern is to produce a see-at-a-glance record which will enable progress to be identified quickly. Figure 9.3 shows one such format which a nurse researcher developed from research on stoma appliance management (Ewing 1984). The teaching plan for the patient is based on a self-care perspective. Thus the helping methods are progressive, with the nurse acting (A) for the learner in the first instance, teaching her (T) when she is ready, guiding her (G) in her learning, supporting her (S) when she does the procedure and assessing when she is completely self-caring (SC). The left-hand column (guidelines) presents a reminder of the steps in care which are to be taught, while the next column records current details of the prescribed care. The dated columns indicate clearly that on Day 1 the nurse did all the stoma care, and on Days 2 and 3 began teaching the patient. By the sixth day the patient is managing with support, but she has not yet achieved total self-care. If this situation still pertained

ACTIVITY 9.2

In this activity, you will set out to evaluate the teaching you planned and carried out for Activity 8.2. You should carry out the same steps you did for Activity 9.1. In this case, if you will have subsequent contact with your learner, you might like to move on to the next teaching need you identify for him or her. Your needs assessment for the next teaching–learning session is virtually covered by what you have done already in the first assessment and in the evaluation of the learning from your first teaching session. So you can move on to the next planning stage, then to the implementation and finally to the evaluation.

This is an example of the teaching–learning process that should be carried out regularly as an integral part of your nursing practice. You will find as you repeatedly practise the process that you become increasingly efficient, and the process will become less time-consuming as you become more expert.

on the day of discharge, a nursing audit might reveal that the teaching process had not progressed sufficiently. This, then, would be a case for discussion.

WHO NEEDS FEEDBACK?

The discussion in this chapter has stressed the importance of feedback: what it is, why we need it, how to provide it, what to do with it. We have dealt with three aspects:

- Feedback for the learner, which will motivate and guide learning
- Feedback for the teacher, which will indicate strengths and weaknesses, allowing for improvements in teaching and for job satisfaction
- Feedback for managers and health care planners, which will help identify effective use of health teaching and thus inform the planning process.

In the end, if the learner has achieved the objectives set in the planning stage and is able to demonstrate the ability to use health knowledge to analyse his or her health problems and potential, to adopt behaviours which promote optimum living, and to hold positive attitudes about such behaviour, then the teaching process may be deemed effective.

However, if the objectives have not been achieved, the evaluation may help to determine the reasons, and the process of teaching begins again with an assessment which may change the plans and actions of the participants so that health teaching becomes an effective tool in the promotion of healthy living.

REFERENCES

Bastable S 2003 Nurse as Educator: Principles of teaching and learning for nursing practice, 2nd edn. Jones and Bartlett Publishers, Sudbury, Massachusetts.

Bloom BS, Hastings JT, Madaus GF 1971 Handbook on formative and summative evaluation of student learning. McGraw-Hill, Toronto.

Boore J 1978 Prescription for recovery. Royal College of Nursing, London.

Cohen D, Hale J 2002 Using economics in health promotion. In: Bunton R, Macdonald G (eds) Health promotion: Disciplines, diversity and developments, 2nd edn, pages 178-96. Routledge, London.

Culyer AJ (ed) 1983 Health indicators: an international study for the European Science Foundation. Martin Robertson, Oxford.

Ewing G 1984 A study of the post-operative nursing care of stoma patients during appliance changes. Unpublished doctoral dissertation, University of Edinburgh.

Green LW 1974 Toward cost benefit evaluations of health education: some concepts methods and examples. Health Education Monographs 2 (Suppl.): 36-64.

Green LW 1977 Evaluation and measurement: some dilemmas for health education. American Journal of Public Health 67(2): 155-161.

Guilbert JJ 1977 Educational handbook for health personnel. World Health Organization Offset Publications No 35, Geneva.

Hayward J 1975 Information: a prescription against pain. Royal College of Nursing, London.

Naidoo J, Wills J 2000 Health promotion: foundations for practice, 2nd edn. Ballière Tindall, London.

Roberts L, Little P, Chapman J, Cantrell T, Pickering R, Langridge J 2002 The back home trial: General practioner-supported leaflets may change back pain behavior. Spine 27(17): 1821-8.

Russell CL, Brown K 2002 The effects of information and support on individuals awaiting cadaveric kidney transplantation. Progress in Transplantation 12(3): 201-7.

ISSUES IN HEALTH TEACHING

10 Research in health teaching

The purpose of this chapter is to address ideas about research relevant to teaching for health, and to introduce some examples of actual research in this area. Box 10.1 contains a selection of journals that should be helpful for carrying out the suggested activities, and for the reader's general use in becoming acquainted with research literature relevant to teaching for health.

ARGUMENTS ABOUT VALUE AND EFFICACY

Health educators and health promoters are convinced of the value of their efforts. They believe that health education and health promotion activities enhance the level of health of individuals and the society they live in. This view is not universally accepted, however, and cynics offer a number of questions to challenge it. Some of these will be touched on in Chapter 11, but one will be addressed specifically in this chapter: the question of the value of health education and promotion activities in terms of their efficacy. That is, do such activities do any good? Are they effective in achieving what they set out to achieve? In the specific case of teaching for health, there are two levels within this question. First, does the teaching lead to learning? And second, does the learning lead to better health?

It may seem to those involved in such activity, or involved more broadly in health care, that the answers to such questions are self-evidently positive: of course health education achieves useful results and is worth doing. But on closer inspection it becomes obvious that the answers are not self-evident, particularly for some types of activities.

In some areas of health teaching, there seems little room to question efficacy and value. When the newly diagnosed diabetic is taught about his disease and

BOX 10.1   *Some useful journal titles*

There are a number of journals whose primary focus is health education or health promotion, and which contain a high proportion of articles related to research. These include:

Health Education Journal. This is published in England by the Health Education Authority. (ISSN 0017 8969)

Health Bulletin. This journal is issued by the Chief Medical Officer of the Scottish Office Home and Health Department. (ISSN 0017 8969)

Health Education Research. This is an international journal published in Britain by the Open University Press. (ISSN 0268 1153)

International Electronic Journal of Health Education. This is published by the American Association of Health Education. (ISSN 1529 1944)

Research in Nursing and Health. This international journal, published in the USA, focuses on research, though not always in health education/promotion. (ISSN 0160 6891)

International Quarterly of Community Health Education. This journal is published in the USA. (ISSN 0272 684X)

Journal of School Health. This is published by the American School Health Association. (ASIN B00006KKPK)

American Journal of Preventive Medicine. This is the journal of the American College of Preventive Medicine and the Association of Teachers of Preventive Medicine. (ISSN 0749 3797)

American Journal of Public Health. This journal has been published since 1911 by the American Public Health Association. (ISSN 0090 0036, E-ISSN 1541 0048)

Several of the well-known journals in nursing and related health care fields occasionally publish articles relevant to health teaching. Most of them may be known to you already:

Nursing Times. A familiar British journal. (ISSN 0954 7762)

Nursing Standard. Another familiar British journal, published in cooperation with the Royal College of Nursing. (ISSN 0029 6570)

American Journal of Nursing. The oldest nursing journal in the world, this is the official journal of the American Nurses' Association. (ISSN 0002 936X, E-ISSN 1538 7488)

Journal of Advanced Nursing (JAN). An international journal, published in Britain, with a more 'academic' flavour than either of the first two. (ISSN 0309 2402, online ISSN 1365 2648)

International Journal of Nursing Studies. Another British journal of similar 'academic' status to JAN. (ISSN 0020 7489)

Sociology of Health and Illness. A British journal of medical/health care sociology. (ISSN 0141 9889, online ISSN 1467 9566)

BMJ. Formerly called the British Medical Journal. (ISSN 0959 8146)

Quality in Health Care. Some articles in this journal, which is published by the BMJ, relate to studies in health education or health promotion.

how to control it, including the testing of urine and blood, the injecting of insulin, and the nutritional and hygienic ramifications, the results are clearly of benefit to the individual's health. Few would quarrel with this. Similarly, the patient who is taught how to manage her colostomy, the father who is taught how to protect his epileptic daughter when she has a fit, the mother who is taught how to prepare a special diet for a family member with a metabolic disease – all these are instances of teaching–learning activities with virtually indisputable value and potential efficacy, if conducted well.

However, there are many areas of health teaching where the results are not so clear cut. When a health visitor, community education worker, or school teacher conducts a session on human relationships and sexuality with a group of young people, it may not be easy to demonstrate the effects of the teaching. There are several reasons for this. It may be straightforward to test the acquisition of cognitive knowledge, but it is virtually impossible accurately to measure the results in terms of behaviour or attitudes. This is particularly true when the impact of teaching has ongoing implications, or implications that will not have an impact until the distant future. Thus, in such cases, even if any measurement can be made, it would be inappropriate to make it immediately following the teaching–learning activity, which is likely to be the only time the health teacher has access to the learners. Even if it is possible to contact the learners at a point in the future, a further complication arises because of the existence of other intervening variables. For the example given above, an individual's success or otherwise in establishing positive relationships and maintaining healthy sexual practices ten years after the teaching–learning episode can prove nothing about the health teaching itself, because many other factors will have influenced the person's attitudes, knowledge and behaviour meantime. So how can the influence of a particular session, or even a whole course, be singled out? The answer is that sometimes it cannot be, at least not with 'scientific' accuracy. However, it is possible to go some way towards identifying the impact of such health teaching activities.

RESEARCHING HEALTH TEACHING

One answer to the challenge regarding the value and efficacy of health teaching is to cite research results in support of its effectiveness. It is evident from the previous discussion that this can be problematic, but there are a number of ways of designing research studies to address the issue. Such studies can be classified into various systems of categorization, or taxonomies. For instance, they can be categorized according to the health topic, or according to the perspective or scope of the study, or according to the type of research method(s) employed in the design. These taxonomies or systems are not separate, of course, and any given study will fall into at least one category within each classification system. Thus, a study can be described as being on a particular health topic, taking a certain perspective, and using a specific method (or more than one) within the research design.

| BOX 10.2 | *Research articles on three health teaching topics* |

Research on the effects of teaching prior to surgery or other procedures:

Mitchell M 2000 Psychological preparation for patients undergoing day surgery. *Ambulatory Surgery* 8(1): 19-29

Mordiffi S Z, Tan S P, Wong M K 2003 Information provided to surgical patients versus information needed. *AORN Journal.* 77(3):546-9, 552-4, 556-8

Shrestha S, Poulos A 2001 The effect of verbal information on the experience of discomfort in mammography. *Radiography* (London) 7(4): 271-7

Webb C 1983 Teaching for recovery from surgery. In: Wilson-Barnett J (ed) *Patient teaching: Recent Advances in Nursing 6.* Churchill Livingstone, Edinburgh

Wilson-Barnett J 1983 Keeping patients informed. *Nursing* 31: 1357-1358

Research on smoking cessation programmes and other related studies:

Altman D G, Flora J A, Fortmann S P, Farquhar J W 1987 The cost-effectiveness of three smoking cessation programs. *American Journal of Public Health* 77: 162-165

Bolman C, deVries H, van Breukelen G 2002 Evaluation of a nurse-managed minimal-contact smoking cessation intervention for cardiac inpatients. *Health Education Research* 17(1): 99-116

Groner J, Ahijevych K, Grossman L, Rich L 1998 Smoking behaviors of women whose children attend an urban pediatric primary care clinic. *Women & Health* 28(2): 19-32

Lennox A S, Bain N, Taylor R J, McKie L, Donnan P T, Groves J 1998 Stages of Change training for opportunistic smoking intervention by the primary health care team – Part 1: randomised controlled trial of the effect of training on patient smoking outcomes and health professional behaviour as recalled by patients. *Health Education Journal* 57(2): 140-9

Macleod Clark J, Haverty S, Kendall S 1989 Communication and health education in nursing: exploring the nurse's role in helping patients and clients to give up smoking. In: Wilson-Barnett J, Robinson S (eds) *Directions in nursing research.* Scutari, London

Rowe K, Macleod Clark J 1993 Evaluating the effectiveness of the coronary care nurses' role in smoking cessation. In: Wilson-Barnett J, Macleod Clark J (eds) *Research in health promotion in nursing.* Macmillan, Basingstoke

Schofield P E, Hill D J, Johnston C I, Streeton J A 1999 The effectiveness of a directly mailed smoking cessation intervention to Australian discharged hospital patients. *Preventive Medicine* 29(6 part 1):527-34

Research on health teaching in schools:

Keirle K, Thomas M 2000 The influence of school health education programmes on the knowledge and behaviour of school children towards nutrition and health. *Research in Science & Technological Education* 18(2): 173-90

McBride N, Midford R 1999 Encouraging schools to promote health: impact of the Western Australian School Health Project. *Journal of School Health* 69(6): 220-6

McIntyre L, Belzer E G Jr, Manchester L, Blanchard W, Officer S, Simpson A C 1996 The Dartmouth Health Promotion Study: a failed quest for synergy in school health promotion. *Journal of School Health* 66(4): 132-7

Munodawafa D, Marty P J, Gwede C 1995 Effectiveness of health instruction provided by student nurses in rural secondary schools of Zimbabwe: a feasibility study. *International Journal of Nursing Studies* 32(1): 27-38

Wiley D C 1993 Training, perceptions and practices of elementary educators regarding health instruction. *Journal of Health Education* 24(3): 169-73

Wong T, Travers K 1998 Evaluation of a peer health education project in The Gambia, West Africa. *International Quarterly of Community Health Education* 17(1): 43-56

Health topics in research

A dip into the literature will reveal that a variety of health topics are addressed in studies of health teaching. A few examples include:

- The effects of teaching prior to surgery or other procedures
- The impact of health teaching strategies on smoking behaviour
- The effectiveness of health teaching in schools.

Several references for each of these areas are offered in Box 10.2. There are, of course, as many potential topics for research as there are topics for health teaching.

The perspectives of health education studies

Researchers in health education or health promotion may approach their topics from different vantage points. Some look at health teaching initiatives or issues within a local, fairly small scope, such as:

- A nutrition teaching project with a primary school class
- A teaching programme to encourage regular physical exercise, carried out on a one-to-one basis with individual overweight patients in a hospital ward
- Teaching of assertiveness skills to disadvantaged women within the case load of an individual health visitor.

Other studies are concerned with the larger picture. Examples of these might include:

- A study of smoking behaviour among staff and patients at all hospitals within the area of a health authority or health board that has adopted a blanket no-smoking policy supported by educational publicity
- A nationwide study of the incidence of road traffic accidents following a media campaign publicizing the links between drinking and driving
- A study of drug misuse among teenagers throughout a region in which the education department has introduced a drugs component into the curriculum for all students in its secondary schools.

Both types of studies are valuable. The government, which must have concern for the value to society of the health education and health promotion campaigns which it funds, may be most impressed by studies with a broad perspective. Professionals, and those involved with education and standards within the professions, may be more interested in studies that address effectiveness at the level of the individual or local group.

Research methods used in health education studies

No serious attempt will be made here to provide a comprehensive account of research methods. Box 10.3 contains suggestions of useful research texts which the reader may wish to consult. A wide range of methods and approaches may be appropriate to research in health education or health promotion, depending on the purpose and context of the research. The following are a few hypothetical examples of research that might be conducted across the range of available approaches:

BOX 10.3	*Useful texts on research method in nursing, education and related social science*

Abbott P, Sapsford R 1998 *Research methods for nurses and the caring professions*, 2nd edn. Open University Press, Buckingham

Balnaves M, Caputi P 2001 *Introduction to quantitative research methods: an investigative approach*. Sage, London

Black T R 1999 *Doing quantitative research in the social sciences: an integrated approach to research design, measurement and statistics*. Sage, London

Bowling A 1997 *Research methods in health: investigating health and health services*. Open University Press, Buckingham

Bryman A, Burgess R G (eds) 1994 *Analyzing qualitative data*. Routledge, London

Buckledee J, McMahon R (eds) 1994 *The research experience in nursing*, Chapman & Hall, London

Cohen L, Manion L 1994 *Research methods in education*, 4th edn. Croom Helm, London

Darlington Y, Scott D 2002 *Qualitative research: stories from the field*. Open University Press, Buckingham

Denscombe M 1998 *The good research guide for small-scale social research projects*. Open University Press, Buckingham

Dey I 1993 *Qualitative data analysis: a user-friendly guide for social scientists*. Routledge, London

Flick U 1998 *An introduction to qualitative research*. Sage, London

Huff D 1954 *How to lie with statistics*. Penguin, Harmondsworth

Knapp T R 1998 *Quantitative nursing research*. Sage, London

Moch S D, Gates M F (eds) 2000 *The researcher experience in qualitative research*. Sage Publications Inc, Thousand Oaks, California

Morse J M, Field P A 1996 *Nursing research: the application of qualitative approaches*, 2nd edn. Chapman & Hall, London

Powney J, Watts M 1987 *Interviewing in educational research*. Routledge, London

Rowntree D 1981 *Statistics without tears: a primer for non-mathematicians*. Penguin, London

Smith P 1997 *Research mindedness for practice: an interactive approach for nursing and health care*. Churchill Livingstone, New York, Edinburgh

Strauss A, Corbin J 1998 *Basics of qualitative research*, 2nd edn. Sage, Thousand Oaks, California

Streubert H J, Carpenter D R 1995 *Qualitative research in nursing: advancing the humanistic imperative*. J B Lippincott Company, Philadelphia

Taylor S J, Bogdan R 1998 *Introduction to qualitative research methods: a guidebook and resource*, 3rd edn. John Wiley & Sons, Inc, New York

Williams F, Monge P R 2001 *Reasoning with statistics: how to read quantitative research*, 5th edn. Harcourt College Publishers, Fort Worth, Texas

See also the references at the end of this chapter.

- A *questionnaire survey* of diabetic patients or clients within a particular health authority or health board area, designed to identify the sources of health teaching they had been exposed to and the extent of their knowledge of matters related to their disease condition
- A *longitudinal study* of young people's attitudes towards drugs, conducted through individual and group interviews carried on over a 5-year period with the same panel of subjects

ACTIVITY 10.1

In this activity, you will explore the literature about a particular health teaching topic. You may approach this in one of two ways:

- Use one of the topics that are given as examples in Box 10.2 and obtain and read the references that are listed for that topic

- Select a health topic that is of interest to you, and locate and read three or four articles that address it.

As you search for literature, you may discover that many of the items you find in doing a key word search do not focus on research about health teaching activities. Some will be about the health problem itself, and others will be 'how-to-do-it' articles about health teaching. These may, of course, be useful for you for other purposes, but not what you are seeking for this activity.

In your search, make full use of the services of your library. It will probably have on-line computer search facilities that will let you get into appropriate databases such as CINAHL (Cumulative Index to Nursing and Allied Health Literature) or ERA (Educational Research Abstracts), and it may also have its own index of articles on specific titles. Remember to take advantage of the library's most useful source of help: the librarian. If you discover that you have chosen an impossible topic and can find no research reports on teaching in that area, switch to another topic.

- An *ethnographic study* of men's perceptions of their own health, involving *participant observation* of a well-man group

- A *randomised controlled trial* of the effectiveness of an innovative teaching initiative for new mothers setting out to breast-feed, comparing their subsequent breast-feeding success with that of a control group taught in the traditional way

- A study of smoking *trends* in relation to a media-based anti-smoking campaign, based on statistical data on tobacco sales in the geographic area exposed to the campaign

- A *historical study* of community health promotion activities, using documentary evidence from the archives of relevant government and non-government agencies, as well as material from the written media.

The above examples suggest single-method studies, but many studies entail the use of a variety of methods. The study of men's perceptions of their health, for example, might also include a questionnaire survey of the same population or a larger population. It might include interviews with individuals or groups of men. The study could be expanded to include an 'oral history' perspective, based on interviews with older men in which their views and memories of how things were in their younger years were explored.

ACTIVITY 10.2

Consider the articles you located for Activity 10.1. For each, identify its perspective. What was the purpose of the study, and do you think the perspective taken was the best for the purpose? Why, or why not? Can you think of other ways in which the topic could be approached, to complement the existing study?

Now, for each of your articles, identify the type of research method or methods that were used. How might other methods have been used to explore this topic, particularly in relation to the additional approaches you identified above?

EVALUATING RESEARCH APPROACHES

Just as health teaching needs to be evaluated, research studies themselves must be evaluated for their credibility and appropriateness. Sometimes the easiest studies to design, and the most convenient ways to take measurements, are not the best or most accurate ways of studying the meaningful effects of a health teaching initiative. For example, it may be quite easy to draw up a questionnaire consisting of true-or-false questions to test cognitive learning, but the acquisition of facts may not be the best indicator of effective learning. The desired learning may not be confined to cognitive knowledge, and affective and psychomotor skills learning cannot be assumed by the learning of relevant factual material.

In addition, the facts that are most readily accessible to an 'objective' type of testing tend to represent low-level or surface-level learning, in cognitive terms: they require primarily recognition and recall. Such learning may not be the most important knowledge to be learned. It may be more important to know if the learner is capable of explaining, analysing, evaluating, problem solving: that is, higher or deep-level learning. The implication of this is that such a means of researching the effects of a health teaching initiative may not be evaluating it in a very meaningful way, and so the research findings may be misleading.

Take the example of a newly diagnosed diabetic. Correct answers on a questionnaire consisting of true-or-false items may tell the researcher (or the teacher) that the individual knows certain facts about blood sugar levels, dietary issues, insulin dosage calculation, and so forth. However, these answers will not show whether the individual can draw up and inject insulin safely, or will adopt a healthy lifestyle based on the learned facts, nor will they indicate whether the individual is capable of problem solving when unanticipated circumstances arise. Thus, a research study making use of such a questionnaire for data gathering will give only a superficial picture of the success of the teaching.

Often the most useful studies for exploring the effectiveness of health teaching make use of more than one research approach, in order to cast light on different aspects of the intended learning. It can be particularly helpful if the combination of methods contains both quantitative and qualitative elements; that is, elements which entail specified measurements that can be counted, such as answers to 'objective' questions or data in a census report, and elements which entail more personal, subjective accounts. In addition, a variety of tech-

ACTIVITY 10.3

Plan a hypothetical research study of your own, to evaluate the effectiveness of a particular (either real or hypothetical) instance of health teaching on a topic of your choice.

First define your health topic and describe the related teaching initiative whose success you would set out to evaluate. Then plan the approach you would take, and the method or methods you would use. Would you study individuals or small groups of people? If so, how would you identify the people or groups? Or would you study the whole population of a community? If so, how would you define the community – based on geography, disease, class, age, gender, or what? Or would you need to use documentary sources? If so, what would they be?

What type of data would you collect, and how would you obtain the data? Would you use questionnaire, interview, observation? How would you analyse the data to enable you to evaluate the success of the teaching initiative? How complete a picture would this give you? What would you do with the findings of the study?

niques may be used for collecting data, including, for example, questionnaires, interviews and observation.

A particular type of research design which may be appropriate for evaluating health teaching initiatives is an approach known as 'action research'. This approach entails collecting data to describe the problem or situation that exists, using this data as a basis for decisions for planning the action or initiative, and then monitoring the effects of the action as it is implemented, using qualitative and quantitative means as appropriate. As the action is monitored, it is adjusted or modified to improve its effectiveness, until the desired outcomes are shown to be resulting from the action.

The similarity between the action research process and the teaching–learning process described in Chapters 6 through 9 is obvious. The needs assessment stage in the teaching–learning process is well suited to the first stage of action research, and the planning and implementation that follow carry on the similarity. The action research notion of continuous evaluation occurring simultaneously with implementation, and serving as feedback to influence further implementation, is similar to the notion of formative evaluation in the education process.

RESEARCH-MINDEDNESS AND THE HEALTH TEACHER

This chapter has focused primarily on research that sets out to evaluate the effectiveness of health education or health promotion activities. Clearly, this is not the only type of research that is useful to the nurse or midwife acting as health teacher.

As in all their professional activities, health teachers have a responsibility to be alert for research findings that are relevant to their area of practice. This is critical to the quality of the content of their teaching. They also need to keep abreast of findings that relate to the phenomena of learning and teaching.

In addition, health teaching activities must be informed by research findings related to health problems and issues. Such research provides part of the basis from which health teaching needs can be identified, targets or goals set, and initiatives planned, particularly from a community perspective. For instance, epidemiological studies which demonstrate the extent of a health problem thereby provide an indication of the amount and type of health education or health promotion effort that should go into addressing that problem. The findings of studies that investigate the effects of health policy can suggest areas for health education in relation to need for empowerment, advocacy, and other community development or political action initiatives.

As a consumer of research, the health teacher needs to be alert and critical. This is especially important in relation to findings that are reported through the public media. When a newspaper headline reads, 'Smoking can be beneficial, say scientists', or 'Junkies reject AIDS warnings', the astute health teacher will be aware that the headline is meant to sell papers and is likely to be a bit light on accuracy. The fine print in the first article may reveal that a (hypothetical) report has found that smoking can be relaxing for people with terminal cancer. A careful reading of the second article may reveal that drug users under age 16, in the community studied, were found to be sharing needles despite health education efforts, but the vast majority of users were consistently using a needle exchange programme. Even then, the careful reader must realize that the article was written by a journalist, and may not represent a full picture of the findings.

The nurse or midwife involved in health teaching needs to operate from a well-informed base, and needs to be secure in the knowledge, skills and attitudes he or she seeks to pass on to clients or patients. To achieve this, it is essential for the health teacher to keep up-to-date with the relevant professional literature.

This chapter has offered only a brief account of research as it applies to health teaching. Readers should refer to texts that specifically focus on research for details about methods and about critical appraisal of research studies. Useful resources include general texts on research methods (e.g. Polit et al 2001), texts that focus on specific types of methods (e.g. Peat et al 2002 for quantitative methods, Denzin & Lincoln 2003 for qualitative methods) or texts specifically about research in health education or promotion (e.g. Oliver & Peersman 2001). A more extensive selection of texts can be found in Box 10.3.

REFERENCES

See Boxes 10.1, 10.2 and 10.3

Denzin NK, Lincoln YS 2003 Strategies of qualitative inquiry, 2nd edn. Sage, Thousand Oaks California.

Oliver S, Peersman G, eds 2001 Using research for effective health promotion. Open University Press, Buckingham.

Peat JK, Mellis C, Williams K, Xuan W 2002 Health service research: a handbook of quantitative methods. Sage, London.

Polit DF, Beck CT, Hungler BP 2001 Essentials of nursing research: methods, appraisal, and utilization, 5th edn. Lippincott, Philadelphia.

11 Reflections on teaching for health

The purpose of this chapter is to address a number of specific issues which are important to teaching for health, but which were not dealt with in depth in the first ten chapters of the book, or were mentioned but are worthy of revisiting.

SUCCESS IN HEALTH TEACHING: ETHICAL AND POLITICAL CONSIDERATIONS

Ethical issues of autonomy and choice

In various places throughout the previous chapters, it has been stated or implied that teaching cannot be said to have occurred unless learning has taken place, and that learning is evidenced by the adoption of a desired behaviour. In one sense, this seems a straightforward position to take. If a driving instructor is trying to teach a student driver to change gears, and after the lesson the student cannot change gears properly, the instructor has not succeeded in teaching the student to change gears. Similarly, if a nurse sets out to teach a patient how to expel air from a syringe when drawing up insulin for injection, and following the lesson the patient is unable to expel air from a syringe of insulin, the teaching has not yet been successful.

In another sense, though, such a position is not straightforward at all. The driving instructor might also hope to impart an attitude of respect for other road users, but how can he or she be sure this has been accomplished? And if the newly licensed driver, who was previously the learner, subsequently does not show respect for other road users, does this necessarily imply that he or she was inadequately taught? At the simplest level, one may conclude that the teaching was unsuccessful in this regard, whatever its quality as an activity. The nurse who is teaching insulin injection may also hope to impart an attitude of acceptance of the need for monitoring sugar levels and administering insulin accordingly. But if the new diabetic does not take these aspects of his or her disease control to heart, is it necessarily the fault of the teaching? Again, one may conclude, at the simplest level, that the teaching was not successful in this respect, whether or not the teaching was competent.

The 'simplest level' is too shallow a level for an analysis of this type, however. It fails to take into account the multitude of other factors that may influence the outcomes of learning, especially in the longer term. The newly qualified driver and the newly diagnosed diabetic both start with feelings, personalities, opinions, values and attitudes of their own. As time goes on, they are both subject to family, peer, financial and advertising pressures, to name a few. They are both capable of being distracted by other stimuli and interests. Thus any learning, whether it relates to health or another sphere of interest, is not a simple product of deliberate teaching activities. Not all good teaching leads to good learning, and not all inadequate learning is attributable to poor teaching. (The reverse is also true, of course: not all poor teaching leads to inadequate learning, and not all good learning is attributable to good teaching.)

It therefore behoves the health teacher to consider other factors that may be at work in the case of the individual learner. Clearly, this should be a concern during the needs assessment (see Chapter 6), but not all such factors will be evident at the time the teaching is planned, and those that are evident may not all be surmountable by good teaching. An important issue in this respect is the ethical right of autonomy of the individual.

Autonomy is the right of the individual to self-determination (see e.g. Doxiadis 1996; Seedhouse 1998; Thompson et al 2000). In behaviour related to health, being autonomous means being able to make one's own choices about how to live one's life. The notion of autonomy has implications in two directions for the health teacher. On one hand, individual autonomy implies the right to make unhealthy lifestyle choices. So if a person with coronary artery disease has learned the dangers of smoking, he nonetheless has the right to choose to smoke. (The issue of passive smoking, and hence the autonomous rights of others, is clearly relevant here, but is another argument.) The individual may care more about the pleasure he gains from smoking, a lifestyle he enjoys, than he does about the prospect of untimely death or disability.

The case suggested above contains the nub of the other angle on autonomy for the health teacher: autonomy cannot be exercised without adequate knowledge. In other words, a person who does not have full information cannot make an informed decision. If the smoker with coronary artery disease does not have a clear understanding of the effects of smoking, he cannot be said to have made an autonomous choice; his decision is limited by insufficient knowledge, so he is not in full control of his choice.

What do these considerations mean in practical terms for the health teacher? For one thing, health teachers have to accept that however strongly they may feel about the content of their teaching, they cannot impose the relevant behaviour on their learners. They have to accept the learners' right to make autonomous choices about their own lifestyle (always assuming that those choices do not infringe other people's rights to autonomy). At the same time, if a learner is to be enabled to make fully competent autonomous choices, the health teacher has a responsibility to ensure that the learner possesses accurate and adequate information. So the notion of autonomy, while it does limit the extent of the health teacher's influence on learners' lifestyles, in no way absolves the teacher from the responsibility to carry out competent teaching.

A number of sources offer useful discussion of ethics related to aspects of health teaching and these offer a fuller discussion of such matters. Examples include Parker (1999), Bradley and Burls (2000), Jones (2000) and Cribb and Duncan (2002).

Political issues of autonomy and compliance

There is yet another perspective on the idea of autonomy, one with political ramifications. When a person makes the 'correct' choices based on health teaching, this is referred to as 'compliance'. Ideally, the patient who has had medications prescribed takes them as instructed; the young people who have attended a session on HIV and AIDS either abstain from sexual activity or indulge only in 'safe sex'; the man who has been taught testicular self-examination and the woman who has been taught breast self-examination carry these procedures out regularly; individuals in a population exposed to a media campaign on good nutrition adopt healthy eating habits. That is, these people comply with the health teaching.

A political question that arises in this respect relates to the degree and nature of the government's responsibility for people's health. In simple terms, a government may decide that it either has responsibility for the health of its citizens or it does not. If it decides that it does, this might be for 'noble' reasons associated with the well-being of the citizens, or it might be a mechanism for trying to cut health care costs – a practical reason. In any case, the decision may involve a question of autonomy: Do individuals within the society have the right to make their own lifestyle choices, or does the government have the right to tell them how to behave, even to compel them to behave 'correctly'? In another view, at a more complex level, it might be seen as a question of attribution of cause: is a person's state of health primarily the result of individual lifestyle choices, or is it more the result of environmental structures and influences?

If a government takes the position that it does have some responsibility for the nation's health, but that health is the result of individual lifestyle choices, then it may be justified in saying, 'We will provide information about how to behave healthily; if people then become unhealthy, it is their own fault.' Thus, autonomy becomes a way of crediting the individual with good health and blaming the individual for bad health. This position is often referred to as a 'victim-blaming' stance (see e.g. RUHBC 1989; Macdonald 2002; Rawson 2002; Ewles & Simnett 2003).

On the other hand, a government might take the position that it has responsibility for the nation's health, and that health is influenced by societal structures and other environmental influences. It would then follow that the government's responsibility extends to altering those influences that are beyond the control of the individual. In other words, according to this stance, it is not justifiable to blame individuals, at least not entirely, for the state of their health.

Thus it can be seen that autonomy can be a two-edged sword. It can be seen as a desirable commodity, important for the individual in that it gives him more control over his own life, providing he is empowered to exercise it. On the other hand, it can be seen as a justification for blaming the individual for the circumstances of his own life, a way for society or government to opt out of responsibility for the welfare of individuals. For the health teacher (or the politician, for that matter), this need not be an 'all-or-nothing' proposition. The positive value of autonomy can be a good reason for fostering it, without its being used as an excuse for doing nothing about structural causes of ill health.

Education, empowerment and autonomy

Autonomy can be seen to be a direct goal of education. The notion of education itself assumes that the individual gains something from learning. It would seem futile if that learning were intended only to fill the individual's brain with facts that the person then had no opportunity or liberty to put to use. Some teaching activities are especially geared to empowering the learner and making him or her more capable of exercising his or her autonomy. It is often not sufficient merely to have adequate knowledge about something. Even with a sound base of knowledge, a person may not have the confidence, the opportunity or the freedom to make the decisions necessary to make use of that knowledge.

Take the case of a woman who has learned the principles of good nutrition. She may have a family, and may wish to put those nutritional principles into practice in the way she provides meals for her family, but her ability to do this may be encumbered by a number of factors. These may include: the availability and price of foods within the shopping area accessible to her; her financial circumstances; the attitudes of her husband or partner and her children; the cooking facilities available in her living accommodation. In order for her to be empowered to make choices about what foods she will buy and how she will prepare the meals, she may need more than a sound knowledge of nutritional principles.

The health teacher faced with such a case needs to take account of the limitations imposed by the learner's circumstances. The planning of the teaching event will need to provide the opportunity to address goals that go beyond the acquisition of nutritional knowledge. In some instances, these goals will simply be unrealistic, and this needs to be acknowledged. In other instances, a potential for positive gain may exist. The goals in such a case may encompass elements such as interpersonal skills for use within the family, skills for dealing with government or other agencies, persuasive skills with which to challenge food-store managers, and so on. For some of these goals, an approach involving a community group may be more effective than an individual approach, particularly when the goals involve encounters with official agencies or other organizations. In any case, it is important to remember that the notional possession of autonomy is of little use if the person is or feels unable to exercise that autonomy.

HEALTH TEACHING IN A CHANGING SCENE

The new education: health teaching across the 'branches'

Throughout this book, an attempt has been made to offer examples that cross the various branches or fields of what is broadly referred to as nursing. These

ACTIVITY 11.1

- Step one: Make a list of aspects of your own lifestyle that are unhealthy. For example, do you smoke? Do you sometimes drink to excess? Do you eat an unhealthy diet, take too little exercise, get too little sleep? Do you drive over the speed limit? Do you feel burdened by stresses you cannot cope with? Do you have arguments with family or friends that damage your relationships? See how many similar examples you can think of.

- Step two: Consider the items on the list you have just made. For each item, answer these questions: Why do I live my life this way, when I know it is unhealthy? (You must realize it is unhealthy, or it wouldn't be on your list!) Do I feel that I have it in my power to choose a healthier behaviour instead? If it is not in my power to choose a healthier behaviour, what is it that stands in my way? Is there any way in which I could remove this barrier?

- Step three: Now consider the positive side of your lifestyle. What choices do you make that are healthy? For example, do you get plenty of exercise? Do you eat a healthy diet? Do you avoid unhealthy sexual activity? Do you balance work with leisure activity? Do you eat plenty of fresh fruits and vegetables? See if you can make this list longer than your first!

- Step four: Consider the items in your 'good health' list. Answer these questions about each item: What motivates you or makes it possible for you to behave in this way? Did you have to overcome any obstacles to achieve this aspect of your lifestyle? If so, how did you do that?

- Step five: Finally, compare your answers from steps two and four. Are there ways in which you could transfer your knowledge and insight about the healthy lifestyle elements to the less healthy elements? This might entail exploring the motivations that lie behind the positive behaviours, as well as looking at how you overcame any obstacles to achieve those behaviours.

This exercise should enhance your ability to understand how external forces and internal motivations may influence the lifestyles of patients and clients you encounter.

contexts include nursing of adults with physical illness, nursing of sick children, mental health nursing, nursing of people with learning disabilities, and midwifery. It is worth emphasizing that health teaching is equally relevant in all these areas, for patients or clients, for families, and for other members of the community. Each area has its own perspective, so the points of particular interest or emphasis may vary.

Nursing of adults with physical illness

In the nursing of adults, examples of teaching may relate to both health and illness. Much patient teaching in acute care facilities is geared to needs created by disease or disability, but nurses in hospital need to be equally aware of learning needs relevant to other aspects of health as well. For instance, a patient who is admitted for surgery needs preoperative teaching specific to that surgery and the experience surrounding it, but may also have learning needs about general health issues, either on his or her own behalf or for the benefit of the family. Family members or significant other persons may also have learning needs related to the patient's illness or other general health issues.

The same principles apply outside the acute health care setting, but the balance of priorities is often towards health-related rather than illness-related learning needs. Another way of expressing this is to say that the teaching needed in hospital is likely to be primarily (but not exclusively) in the realms of tertiary prevention, while in the community it may be more in the realms of primary and secondary prevention. In addition, whereas the individual patient is usually the main (but not only) recipient of teaching in hospital, the family and other members of the community may figure more strongly as recipients of teaching in the community setting.

It is probably unwise to see a strict dichotomy between the teaching–learning activities that go on in the acute care setting and those that go on in the community setting. It is more productive to see them as part of the same spectrum, both in general terms and with reference to the individual patient or client. The differences are not absolute but are a matter of emphasis.

Nursing of sick children

The above comments about the nursing care of adults apply to the nursing of sick children, for the most part. There is one apparent major difference, though it may not be as stark as at first appears: children may be too young to be the primary recipients of health teaching. One implication of this is the critical nature of the needs assessment. How ready and able is the child to be responsive to teaching? The answer to this question must depend in part on the developmental stage of the child. Consideration should be given to cognitive, psychomotor and emotional aspects of development. In addition, the health teacher must take into account any impact the present circumstances may have on the child's receptivity. A child who has just been in an accident, or who is in pain following surgery or as a result of illness, or who is frightened by unfamiliar surroundings, is unlikely to be receptive to teaching.

As was indicated above, this feature of health teaching for children appears to be different from the health teaching of adults, but this may be only a matter of degree. Not all adults are capable of being receptive to health teaching, for some of the same reasons. Regarding cognitive ability, the causes of limitation in adults may relate to injury, disease or degeneration, rather than to developmental stage, but the same issues need to be taken into consideration. The other side of this coin, figuratively speaking, is that the health teacher should not underestimate a child's potential for learning. Diabetic children, for example, may be capable of learning to test their own urine or blood and administer their own insulin injections at surprisingly young ages. The same principle can pertain to cognitive and affective learning in children, and it can sometimes be damaging to a child to be told too little, or to be 'protected' from unpleasant knowledge. Children usually benefit from being full participants in learning about their health, to whatever extent they are capable of comprehending.

Mental health nursing

In mental health nursing, the focus of health teaching may be related more to social and emotional health than to physical health. But here again, this apparent difference is often a matter of emphasis or degree rather than being absolute. Thus, while the first priority is likely to be for teaching–learning activities that focus on mental health, the patient or client may have just as much need for teaching about physical health as does a patient or client in any other field of nursing.

It is equally important to remember that patients and clients who are not designated as 'mental' or 'psychiatric' may also have learning needs related to mental health. The issue of mental health is sometimes a problematic one in health education, in that many people conceive of mental health only in relation to mental illness. That is, the notion of mental health is seen as the absence of mental illness or abnormality – conditions such as schizophrenia, clinical depression and obsessional neurosis. This view omits everyday aspects of mental health, such as the building of positive interpersonal relationships, the development of self-esteem, or coping with everyday stress. The latter aspects are relevant to virtually everyone, and thus they may be present as learning needs for patients or clients, family members, and community groups in almost any context that may be imagined.

Nursing of people with learning disabilities

Examples of health teaching abound in the nursing of people with learning disabilities. The broad approach to teaching, that is, teaching aimed at the individual, the family and significant other persons, and the community, can be illustrated by a case example. When a child is born with Down's syndrome, initially the parents and other members of the family circle will need teaching about what to expect. They will need to understand what Down's syndrome is and how it may affect the child, and they will need ongoing advice on the care of the child. They will need to be put in touch with resources that will provide them with appropriate support at various stages in the child's development. As time goes on, the child him- or herself will need teaching. A careful needs assessment will be particularly important, as will the setting of reasonable goals and a sensitive approach to the methods and styles of teaching. Within the community, there is a need for education about Down's syndrome. Public education is needed as to what the syndrome is, and it is particularly important to dispel misunderstandings about the behaviour of people with Down's syndrome. This is an area in which learning within both the cognitive and affective domains is essential. A general understanding that people with Down's syndrome are individuals, with unique personalities, normal human emotions, and a need to feel valued, for example, will enhance the community's ability to be a positive environment, both for the individual with the learning disability and for the community as a whole.

Midwifery

Much of the teaching in midwifery is about health rather than illness or disability, because pregnancy, childbirth and parenthood are normal and usually healthy parts of life's experience. The first recipient of teaching is, of course, the expectant or new mother, with other recipients in a widening circle around her – the woman's partner, siblings of the new baby, grandparents, and so on. Midwifery provides a neat example of the importance of the continuity of health teaching referred to earlier. The midwife participates in clients' care throughout the antenatal, perinatal, and postnatal periods, covering the spectrum in a continuous programme of supportive health teaching.

Some topics that are of specific relevance to midwifery are also relevant in a broad sense to the community – topics such as preconception health, antenatal nutrition and parenting skills. Thus the midwife, like the nurse, may be called upon to undertake health teaching activities that go beyond the specific practice of midwifery.

The shifting focus of care: the move to the community

In the examples given above, of health teaching across the fields of nursing and midwifery, the relevance of teaching in the community is evident. Earlier in this book, reference was made to the significant changes that have been taking place in the National Health Service in the UK in and other countries. These have included features of an increasingly market-based approach to the delivery of health care over the past few years, such as the establishment of purchaser–provider arrangements throughout the system, both for delivery of care and for the education of health care professionals. One element of current health services in many countries is the accelerating emphasis on community care, accompanied by the slimming-down of in-patient services and the centralizing or 'rationalizing' of those services.

For the nurse or midwife acting as health teacher, there are important implications in this shift away from an acute care focus towards community care. For one thing, it can be assumed that in future, proportionately more nurses will be working in the community. Thus many nurses' teaching skills will have to be adapted more to teaching in that setting than to teaching in a clinical setting. This in turn entails another set of implications. The client in the community tends to be less a 'captive audience' than is the hospital patient, with the nurse being a guest in the home or other community context. The nurse working in the community will thus be in a less controlling position, and negotiating skills may become increasingly important. This might be seen as making the nurse's task more difficult or challenging. On the other hand, since the nurse's interaction with the client will be more likely to take place in the client's normal living context, it may be easier to carry out a realistic and effective assessment of learning needs, and thus to plan more effective teaching. In addition, the evaluation of the results of teaching also have the potential to be more realistic, since it will be done in the setting in which the client lives. Further to this point, the breadth of health-related needs may become more apparent, helping the nurse to avoid concentrating excessively on illness-related needs.

Outside the hospital setting, nurses will have to rely more on their own resources, as they may be working in isolation and will not have other staff and sophisticated equipment readily at hand to assist in the teaching task. Here again an apparent disadvantage is counterbalanced by an advantage: clients may experience greater continuity of care and teaching, if they are visited by the same nurse over an extended period of time. In hospital, even with 'primary care' or 'named nurse' systems operating, patients may experience care by a bewildering number of professionals, and nursing staff can find it difficult to ensure that the coherence of the teaching–learning programme provided for an individual patient is maintained.

Another set of important implications of the recent changes relates to the nurse's teaching role in the acute care setting. As more and more care is relocated to the community setting, and hospital stays become shorter, covering only the most critical stages of illness or treatment, the opportunities for health teaching for the individual patient in hospital will inevitably be curtailed. This situation may be exacerbated by changes in the 'skill mix' of clinical staff, with care being delivered by fewer qualified nurses and more unqualified care staff. Thus, the nurse will need to become proficient in setting priorities for teaching and in implementing teaching programmes in a highly efficient manner. Teaching may have to focus largely on immediate illness-related learning needs, with other learning needs being postponed until they can be attended to by a nurse or other health teacher in the community.

There is a challenge inherent in this situation for the profession: to ensure that the learning needs of individuals are met, in both illness-related and health-related aspects. In the scenario just described, this challenge may appear to be difficult to meet, given the limited contact between professional nurses and patients in hospital, and the limited staffing that is perceived to exist at present in the community. It might be argued, however, that the answer is for nurses, and for the profession as a whole, to get rid of outworn conceptions of how nursing care should be implemented, and to rethink some aspects of how the nursing role is formulated.

ACTIVITY 11.2

In the clinical or community area in which you have been working, can you think of instances of health teaching that you have observed taking place between a health teacher and a patient or client? Perhaps you have carried out some health teaching yourself. If possible, list three such examples of health teaching from your recent experience, whether carried out by you or by someone else. For each example, consider the following:

■ What was the teaching topic? Was it health-related or illness-related?

■ Who was the recipient of the teaching? Was it the patient or client, or was it a member of the family or a significant other person, or was it a group?

■ Can you think of additional teaching that might accompany this particular instance? This might be to other recipients, and/or the same recipient at an earlier or later time. Identify this additional teaching as to its time, place and recipient(s).

■ Draw a diagram that represents the interrelated teaching in terms of its recipients, its location (e.g. hospital, home, school classroom) and its chronological order.

Once you have done this exercise for each of your three examples, compare your three diagrams. What does your comparison tell you about the features of health teaching that are similar and those that are individual or specific?

One way of approaching this would be to move away from a view of health teaching as an additional task in the nurse's repertoire, to a view that health teaching is integral to all aspects of the nurse's role. In other words, health teaching would permeate the nurse's role instead of being singled out as a separate task. (This point is addressed again at the end of this chapter.) Although there has been a strong task-based tradition underpinning British nursing practice (Dingwall et al 1988), many nurses and midwives already practise in this more integrated way. Given the enhanced level of nursing and midwifery education following the changes that have taken place in the UK and many other countries during the 1990s, the ability of nurses and midwives to meet this challenge should be similarly enhanced.

PROFESSIONAL INTERFACES

In their professional roles, nurses and midwives come into contact with a wide variety of other professionals and non-professionals who have an interest in health education. Some nurses and doctors hold the view that an activity can only justifiably be called 'health education' if it is carried out by health professionals. This is an excessively narrow and inaccurate view of health education; some might call it arrogant. Teaching related to health goes on almost from the moment a person is born, and it is carried out, whether formally or informally, by parents and other relatives, teachers, neighbours, members of the clergy, television presenters, fellow students – in other words, almost any person seen by the individual to be in a position of authority or 'in the know'. Of course, not all these people see themselves as being health teachers, but it is not only health professionals who do consciously see themselves in that role.

School teachers, for example, have a responsibility for health education. This is explicit in the National Curriculum for England (DFEE 1999), and in the 'Five to Fourteen' curriculum in Scotland (Scottish Executive 2000). In fact, if the WHO's definition of health (see Chapter 1) is accepted, virtually everything that goes under the heading of 'education' is in some sense related to health, and thus all teachers are involved in health education. This is perhaps particularly true of the role of community education workers, whose educational activities with young people tend to be less bound by formal curricula than are those of school teachers.

It is important for nurses and midwives to remember that others who have just as legitimate a role to play may have different views of health education. For instance, while the nurse's view of health education may be based on an amalgam of the medical and educational models, the community worker probably has a view based more on a community development model.

An important implication of this is that nurses need to recognize the legitimacy of health teaching done by individuals outside the health professions. It is true that nurses need to be aware of the potentially negative health messages emanating from, for example, television, Internet or magazine advertising. However, the constructive health teaching carried out by others, and the health teaching carried out by nurses and midwives, are best seen as being complementary to each other. If this view is accepted, then it follows that nurses and midwives should work in cooperation with other such educators.

ACTIVITY 11.3

Recall the exercise you carried out for Activity 11.2. Are there other individuals, either health professionals, professionals from fields other than health, and/or non-professionals, who might also be involved in the health teaching identified in your three examples? Who are they, and when and how might they be/have been involved? Add these individuals to your three diagrams as appropriate.

FINAL REFLECTIONS: THE PLACE OF HEALTH TEACHING IN THE WORK OF NURSES AND MIDWIVES

One premise on which this book is based is that health teaching is a vital part of the role of the nurse or midwife. It is just as important as any other element of care. A final point that needs to be emphasized in relation to this, one that was alluded to earlier, is that health teaching is not an activity separate from nursing care. That is, it should not stand in isolation from the nurse's or midwife's other activities.

This is not to say that there are not times especially given over to teaching, or that there are not activities clearly marked out as teaching. What it does mean is that health teaching should be integrated with the other activities of care.

In some cases, this integration is a practical one. That is, the teaching is done while other aspects of care are being administered. Small instances of teaching may be carried out on-the-spot, as the need becomes obvious – teaching about a newly prescribed medication when it is first administered to a patient in hospital, for example, or reinforcing aspects of safe wound dressing while watching a client change his own dressing at home. In other cases, the teaching may be planned more formally, but may still take place during other care, such as when the nurse whose patient will be having bronchoscopy explains aspects of the procedure to the patient while giving him or her a bath the day before the investigation is to take place.

Some instances of teaching are deliberately planned and carried out as discrete teaching–learning sessions, and therefore stand alone rather than occurring during other care. Such teaching, while it occurs separately from other activities, should nonetheless be conceptually integrated with the rest of the patient's or client's care. For example, a teaching session on stoma care should not be planned to occur until the patient has become able to accept the presence of the stoma.

Thus the nurse or midwife undertaking health teaching should consider how it fits with the patient's or client's overall care. Similarly, nurses and midwives giving care to patients or clients should be constantly alert for the teaching–learning needs and possibilities that relate to that care. Teaching for health should not be *in addition* to patient or client care; it should be *an integral part* of it.

REFERENCES

Bradley P, Burls A (eds) 2000 Ethics in public and community health. Routledge, London.

Cribb A, Duncan P 2002 Health promotion and professional ethics. Blackwell Science, Malden, Massachussetts.

Department for Education and Employment (DFEE) 1999 Curriculum for PSHE. Department for Education and Employment, London.

National Curriculum online: http://www.nc.uk.net/index.html Accessed September 20, 2003.

Dingwall R, Rafferty AM, Webster C 1988 An introduction to the social history of nursing. Routledge, London.

Doxiadis S (ed) 1996 Ethics in health education. Wiley, New York.

Ewles L, Simnet I 2003 Promoting health: a practical guide. Ballière Tindall, Edinburgh

Jones SR 2000 Ethics in midwifery. Mosby, London.

Macdonald G 2002 Communication theory and health promotion. In: Bunton R, Macdonald G (eds) Health promotion: disciplines, diversity and elements, 2nd edn. Routledge, London, pages 196-218.

Parker M (ed) 1999 Ethics and community in the health care professions. Routledge, London.

Rawson D 2002 Health promotion theory and its rational construction: lessons from the philosophy of science. In: Bunton R, Macdonald G (eds) Health promotion: disciplines, diversity and elements, 2nd edn. Routledge, London, pages 249-270.

RUHBC (Research Unit in Behavioural Change, University of Edinburgh) 1989 Changing the public health. Wiley, Chichester.

Scottish Executive 2000 5-14 Guidelines: health education. Scottish Executive, Edinburgh; Learning and Teaching Scotland: http://www.ltscotland.org.uk/5to14/guidelines/ Accessed September 20, 2003.

Seedhouse D 1998 Ethics: the heart of health care. Wiley, Chichester.

Thompson IE, Melia KM, Boyd KM 2000 Nursing ethics, 4th edn. Churchill Livingstone, Edinburgh.

1 Questions for review and reflection

1. How would you define health? Look back at Chapter 1 and see how your definition compares with the definitions given for Activity 1.1.

2. Explain the difference between primary, secondary and tertiary prevention, and give a specific example of each.

3. Discuss the relevance of epidemiology to health education and promotion.

4. Describe an instance in which statistics might help the health teacher to understand a health problem.

5. What health problems do you think are particularly significant in your community? How could you find out more about their extent, and about what is being done to tackle them?

6. In what ways can government policy influence the health of the nation, either for better or for worse? In discussing this, remember to consider not just policies whose purposes are directly related to health, but also those that have other purposes but have an impact on health.

7. Discuss the proposition that the health teacher should not manipulate the client.

8. Describe four models of health education, and discuss the strengths and limitations of each model.

9. Discuss the role of the agency responsible for health education or health promotion in your national area. Find out which local agency has responsibility in your own community. What resources does it offer that you might make use of in your health teaching? (You might like to visit it and see for yourself.)

10. Identify each of the following health teaching situations according to which one or more of the domains of learning it entails, and explain briefly how the domains are involved:

    a. Preoperative preparation for termination of pregnancy
       Domain(s):
       Explanation:

    b. Diabetic teaching with an adolescent involved in sport
       Domain(s):
       Explanation:

c. Self-management teaching with a 60-year-old man with asthma
Domain(s):
Explanation:

d. Teaching 'keep fit' exercises to a group of adolescent girls
Domain(s):
Explanation:

11. Describe the difference between deep-level and surface-level processing in learning, and the difference between serialist and holist approaches to learning. For each pair, discuss the relative effectiveness of the two types of approach for different types of learning tasks, giving examples to illustrate your points.

12. Discuss factors that may affect a person's motivation and readiness to learn.

13. Classify the following as:

■ open-ended questions

■ closed questions

■ leading questions

a. 'Can you tell me more about the feelings you have when you meet with friends in a pub?'

b. 'Where is the pain most severe?'

c. 'Did you enjoy that film?'

d. 'Do you find the smell of your colostomy offensive?'

e. 'What is your day like when you are at home?'

f. 'How long have you felt nervous?'

g. 'Is the meal delicious?'

h. 'Where would you like your injection, the right arm or the left arm?'

In the case of questions you have identified as closed or leading, change their wording to make them open-ended questions. Which is better for the implied purpose of the question?

14. Outline an appropriate health teaching approach for each of the following situations, indicating the methods(s) and audiovisual aids you might use:

a. The wife of an accountant, who has two children at home, is about to be discharged 48 hours after delivery of a healthy baby boy.

b. A 25-year-old female has had recurrent bouts of cystitis since the age of 12 years. She has no symptoms at the moment. She is recently married and has no children.

c. Bus drivers at a local depot have asked the staff of a health promotion department for information about heart disease. A scare report in a newspaper prompted the enquiry.

15. Discuss the factors that might influence your choice of teaching methods and audiovisual aids in the above examples.

16. Prioritize the learning needs of a middle-aged male smoker who suffers from chronic bronchitis and has been admitted to hospital in a very breathless state.

17. Discuss how you would go about assessing the learning needs of a new mother, if you were visiting her and her new baby at home.

18. Rewrite the following objectives so they describe terminal behaviour of the learner and indicate unambiguously the criterion of success:

   a. Know the reasons for including adequate fibre in the diet

   b. Be competent to give an insulin injection

   c. Understand the dangers of HIV.

19. Write a set of objectives likely to meet the initial preoperative teaching needs of a 50-year-old woman undergoing hysterectomy for uterine fibroids.

20. John McWilliam is 72 years old and due to go home from hospital soon. He lives alone, but has an attentive daughter who visits regularly and lives nearby. He has to have three different medications and has become agitated on the two occasions on which his drug regime for home has been discussed. He insists he knows which drugs to take, but members of the nursing staff are uncertain of this. Draw up a plan for teaching.

21. Emma, who is 6 years old, has a badly injured finger. Surgeons wish to operate, to prevent dysfunction. Her parents reject technological medicine and have refused permission. You have been asked to persuade them to give permission for surgery. What factors will influence your chance of success?

22. Discuss the purposes of planned evaluation of health teaching.

23. A health visitor is evaluating her efforts to teach new parents about the importance of play in their children's life. Which one or more of the following techniques would be useful in evaluating the process of teaching and learning, and how might they be used effectively?

   a. Check list

   b. Anecdotal notes

   c. Teacher diary

   d. Written assessment.

24. Debate the proposition that 'teaching for health is a worthwhile activity'. In making your case, as well as using logical argument, use your knowledge of research studies in health education to support your stand either for or against the proposition.

25. Discuss the idea that health education should reduce health care costs.

26. Discuss the place of health teaching in the role of the nurse or midwife.

Index

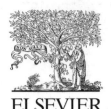

ELSEVIER

 Books *for* **Midwives**

 CHURCHILL LIVINGSTONE   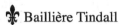 **Mosby**   **THE PRACTISING MIDWIFE**   ✣ **Baillière Tindall**

MIDWIFERY PUBLISHERS OF CHOICE FOR GENERATIONS

For many years and through several identities we have catered for professional needs in midwifery education and practice. Leading publishers of major textbooks such as *Myles Textbook for Midwives* and *Mayes' Midwifery: a Textbook for Midwives*, our expertise spreads across both books and journals to offer a comprehensive resource for midwives at all stages of their careers.

Find out how we can provide you with the right book at the right time by exploring our website, **www.elsevierhealth.com/midwifery** or requesting a midwifery catalogue from Health Professions Marketing, Elsevier, 32 Jamestown Road, Camden, London, NW1 7BY, UK Tel: 020 7424 4200; Fax: 020 7424 4420.

We are always keen to expand our midwifery list so if you have an idea for a new book please contact Mary Seager, Senior Commissioning Editor at Elsevier, The Boulevard, Langford Lane, Kidlington, Oxford, OX5 1GB, UK (m.seager@elsevier.com).

 Have you joined yet?
Sign up for e-Alert to get the latest news and information.

Register for eAlert at www.elsevierhealth.com/eAlert Information direct to your Inbox

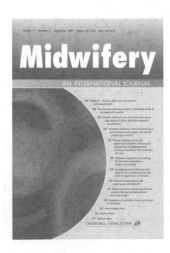

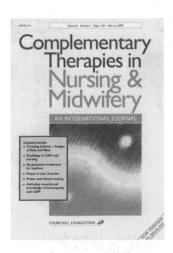